Good for what Ails you

Self-Help Remedies from 19th Century Canada

Jim Cameron

Published by

GSPH GENERAL STORE PUBLISHING HOUSE

1 Main Street, Burnstown, Ontario, Canada K0J 1G0
Telephone 1-800-465-6072 Fax (613) 432-7184

ISBN 0-919431-93-3
Printed and bound in Canada

Layout and Design by Leanne Enright
Cover Design by Tammy Anderson and Eugenia Sagardia

General Store Publishing House gratefully acknowledges the assistance of the Ontario Arts Council and Canada Council.

Canadian Cataloguing in Publication Data

Cameron, James M. (James McIntyre), 1942-

Good for what ails you: self-help remedies from 19th century Canada

ISBN 0-919431-93-3

1. Self-care, Health. 2. Medicine, Popular. I. Title.

RC81.C35 1995 615.8'8 C94-900918-0

First Printing July 1995

To

Helen Althea Ross McIntyre (1878 - 1967)
who trained as a nurse at the end of the
19th century and was the only grandmother whom
I was fortunate enough to know

and

Catherine Margaret Cameron, my daughter
who has tried to promote the health of her father,
sometimes with success.

Table of Contents

Preface

As I suspect is usual in writing a preface, the author somehow manages to finish the book and then, either in exhaustion or joy, tries to think of something else to say. I should state however, that while the following self-help remedies are in a variety of ways interesting, unusual and often practical—the author neither suggests nor warrants their use by any "man (or as some would prefer, person) or beast." Such a disclaimer is made both appropriate and necessary by the increasing lack of personal responsibility for one's own choices and actions, by society's overproduction of lawyers and by the generally poor financial state of most Canadian authors.

The process of writing *Good For What Ails You* has been both an interesting and a learning experience. My first glimpse of 19th century Canada and its social context began in conversations with my adoptive maternal grandfather, Elmer F. McIntyre, who always had a vignette to tell a captive audience—even of one. Beyond this personal contact, the period was also an important part of Canada's social and economic evolution. The sources of information are extensive, in libraries and archives and easily available to anyone with an interest. However, in a real sense, the period is "so close but yet so far." It seems to be within reach, but always slightly out of our grasp or focus.

Writing a book is, by definition, a very personal experience, so I shall let myself expand for a moment on this theme. In gathering information, I wrote to weekly newspapers and Women's Institutes across Canada and received hundreds of responses, unfortunately only some of which I was able to include in the book. In June 1993, Mrs. Dora Rutherford, 85 years young, wrote from her apartment in Orillia, Ontario, with several home remedies which her family had used. She noted that her childhood days had been on the farm in Oro Township. As my father's family had been early settlers in this area, I phoned her and we spoke at some length. Amazingly, she knew my grandfather, who had died before I was born, and my favourite great uncle, Nels Roberts, who she described as "the one with the smiling eyes." One can only imagine my feelings in talking to someone who had personal contacts with these individuals out of my family's past. Such are the unexpected, yet poignant moments, in a project such as this.

The book's theme has uniformly met with interest from friends as well as strangers, who have always been willing to share not only their remembrances, but a variety of other sources of information.

I owe particular thanks to John Dawson who, as usual, has been ready with his camera; John Becker, who is always ready to help a friend; Eugenia Sagardia, whose artistic sensitivity helped design the cover; Ted Jackman, whose company is always enjoyable, particularly when one is searching for UFOs with Tim and Rosemary; Regina Pinto, who has not only suffered through a convoluted collection and inputting process, but has done it with patience, style and good humour; Susan Code whose role as editor has been not only a helpful one, but also one of good taste; and, Leanne Enright whose unsung efforts are much appreciated by the author.

Scrapper, Quibble, Sweet-Pea and their kith'n kin always provided encouragement for the task at hand and served as a constant reminder that every book is different, not just its cover.

Let me also thank Jim, who knows the interlibrary loan system better than most and was willing to help his Luddite father; Cathy, who discovered the extent of the Ontario Archives; Dave, who knows how to operate a microfiche reader-printer; Andrew, who somehow manages to put up with his father's prying questions and Jack, my favourite son-in-law, who secretly wonders why anyone should be paid to do what they really enjoy doing anyway. Finally, Newton (Sir Isaac), although older and wiser, continued to remain somnolent and Kaye, who was normally patient with my untidy mess and constant wanderings in and out of 19th century Canada.

Jim Cameron
Kleinburg, Ontario
June, 1995.

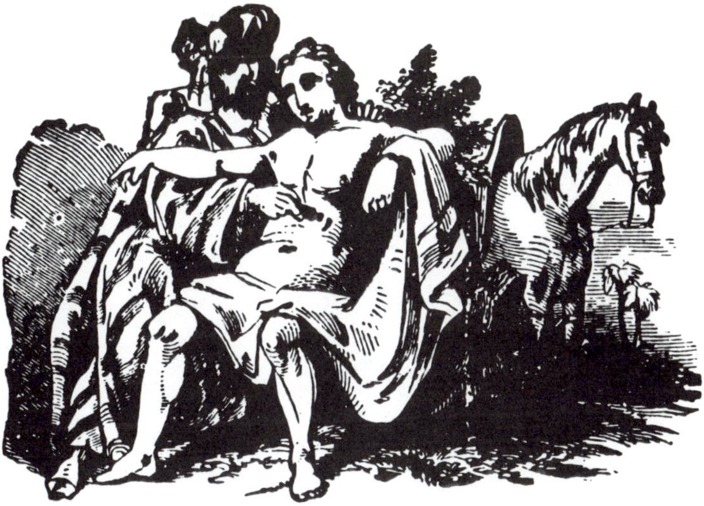

THE GOOD SAMARITAN.

Health and the simplest fare. If thou hast these,
Accompanied with one single steadfast friend—
A conscience which thou dost not fear to bear
To the Great Searcher's eye—and that strong hope
Whose wing ne'er tires, e'en o'er the yawning grave,
Go thou thy way; thou art an emperor,—
Bearing thy crown e'er with thee; go thy way
And thank thy God, who hath bestowed on thee
The gold which monarchs count, but oft in vain.

The *Household Guide*, Toronto, 1894

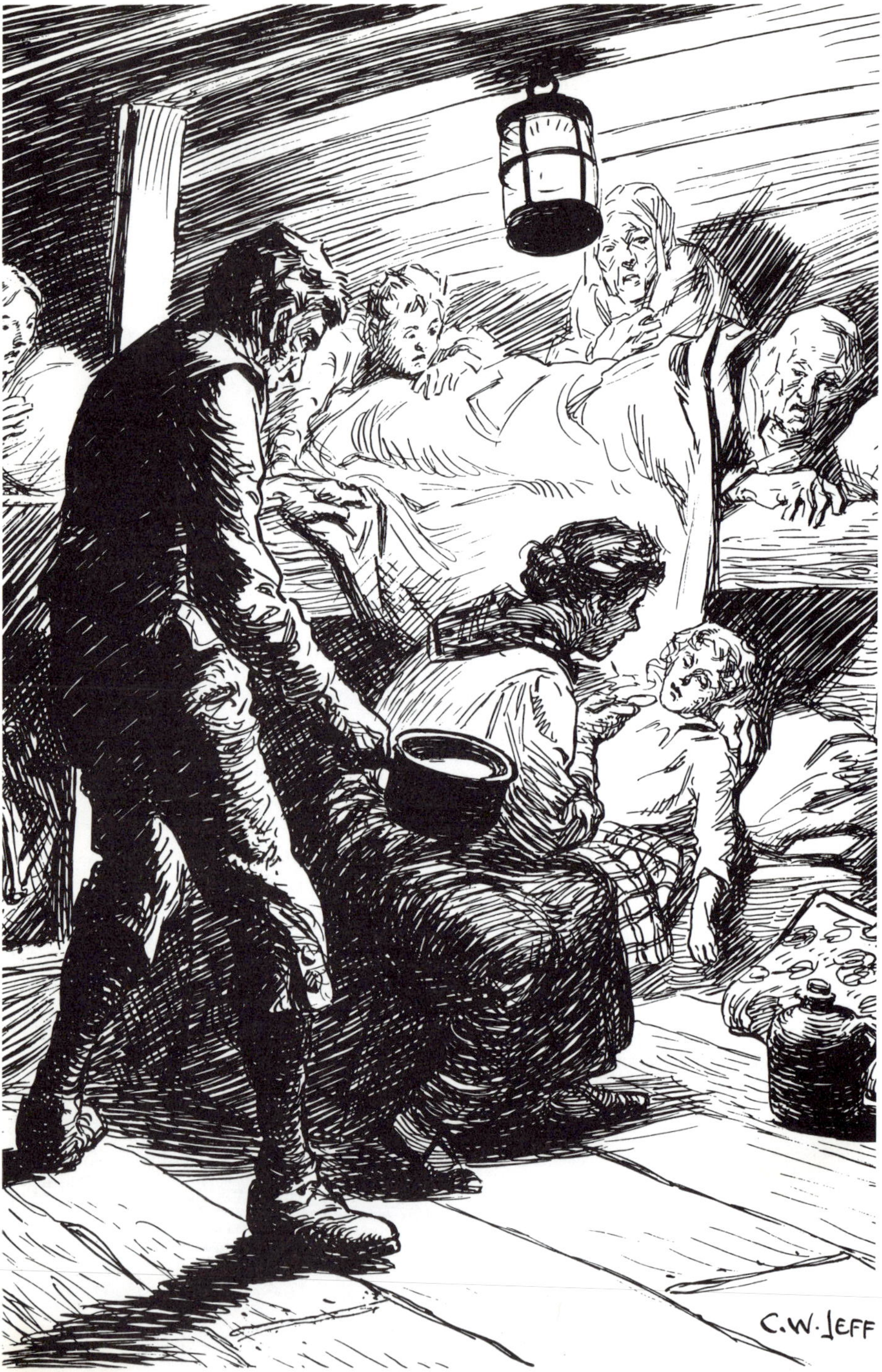

On board an emigrant ship in the thirties, C. W. Jefferys, National Archives of Canada, C73435, with permission of the C. W. Jefferys Estate Archives

Prologue

This book deals with aspects of self-help medicine as presented by 19th century sources in English speaking Canada. There is a wealth of material available dealing with practices by natives and French Canadians of the same period, but neither time nor space afforded the author the opportunity of including this information. Indeed, they deserve their own coverage.

The remedies/receipts/recipes included in *Good For What Ails You* are those which were presented or advocated in books, pamphlets and newspapers of the period. They present a unique, some would say even bizarre, perspective on the social and medical views and values of the time. They cannot, and should not, be taken as anything more or less than a social/cultural vignette of a time which has passed. Yet, self-help medicine had a very considerable status and value during this period—more about this later.

The following brief prologue identifies the role of self-help medicine in its appropriate place within the broader scope of medicine, that is, the provision of cures or treatments for real or perceived ailments and sicknesses. Indeed, medicine in this context has had a long, varied and often complex history, certainly for as long as people have been people and ailments have been ailments.

The migration of thousands, and then tens of thousands, of individuals and families from Europe to North America, beginning in the 17th and 18th centuries, brought with it the traditions and backgrounds of the European experience, largely from the British Isles. The cultural "baggage" which people carried with them, their myths, folk medicine, home cures, specific remedies and the beginnings of professional medicine, all arrived together in North America. Of necessity, they had to be integrated into the new society in which both individuals and families found themselves.

Majority, main stream, regular or, as we would call it today, "professional" medicine, was still evolving. This was the period prior to the clinical and scientific medicine as we know it today. At the time, the use of "extreme measures," such as blood letting, and the use of arsenic

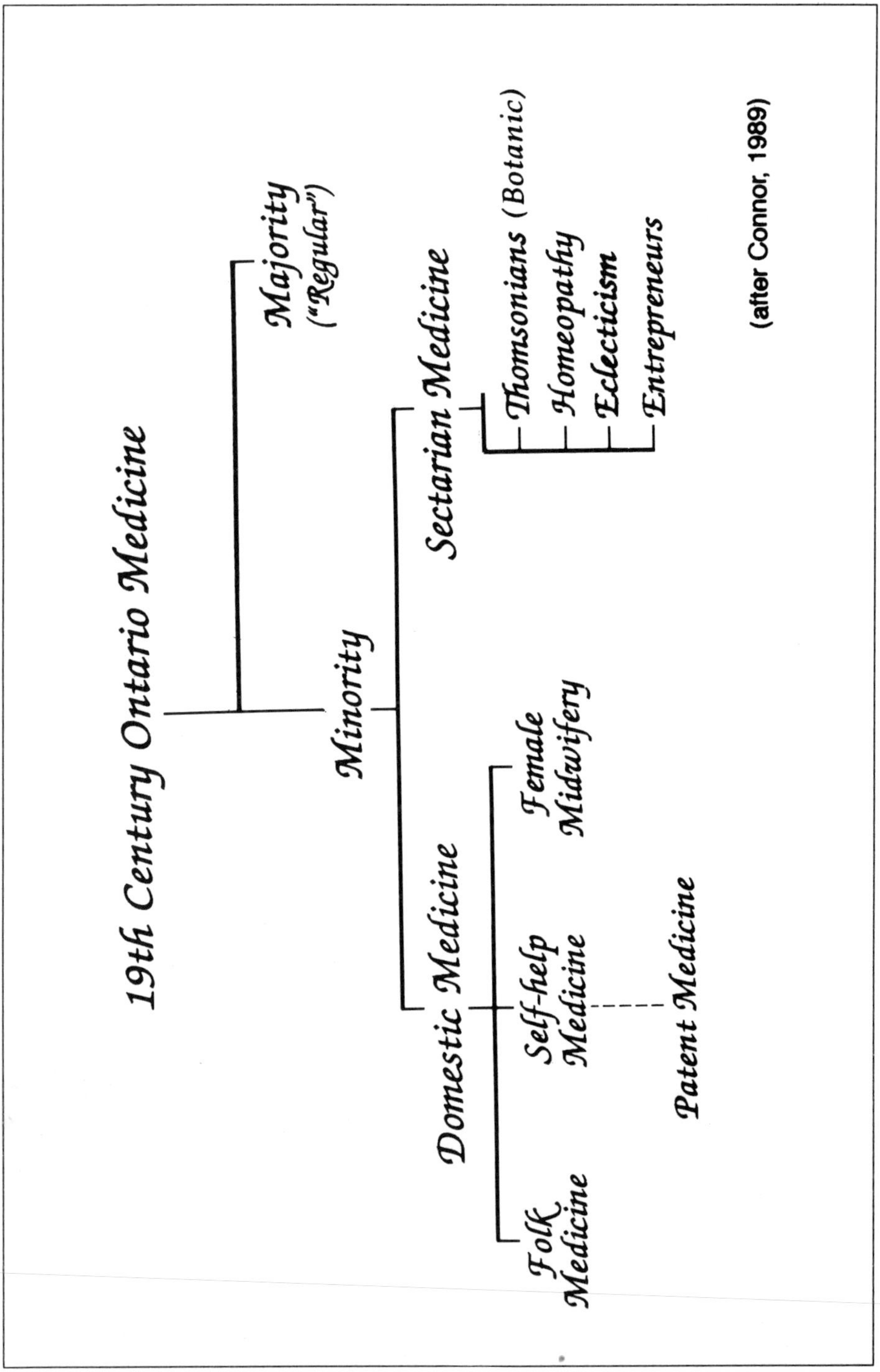

Chart A-19th Century Ontario Medicine

and mercury were commonly used treatments. The medical profession did not have all or even most of the answers and individuals knew that. Indeed, their cures were often much worse than the ailments. During the first half of the 19th century, Canada was only beginning to see the development of a pioneer agricultural society and a nascent urban industrial society. Accessibility to and the costs of mainstream medicine meant that many of these services were not readily available, even if individuals needed them or chose to make use of them.

On the other hand, individuals and communities were not left in a void. Minority medicine broadly defined (see Chart A) consisted of both the traditional provision of domestic medicine as well as various sectarian medical groupings. In this framework, domestic medicine consists of three areas—folk medicine, self-help medicine (including patent medicine) and female midwifery.

Folk medicine refers to an essentially oral tradition of superstitions, myths and images which evolved over many hundreds of years. The curing powers of the seventh son of the seventh son and the hair of a black cat are but two examples of this genre. Such broadly based cultural beliefs continued to have status with individuals and families in many parts of Canada during the 19th century. Although not a central focus of this book, folk medicine is briefly presented as part of the social context of the period.

Self-help medicine in its many and varied forms has always been a part of the human condition. In essence, it is the attempt by individuals, beyond the mythical context of folk medicine, to use, evaluate and pass on particular remedies which were perceived to be "good for what ails you." They were the remedies/cures which families or neighbours had tried and found to be effective in treating particular and often common ailments. They consisted of ingredients which, when combined together or used singly, brought relief or apparent cures for specific problems. If they seemed to have worked, they were passed from one generation to another. In a significant sense, they were a step beyond folk cures because they were specific natural remedies which had been tried and felt to be more effective in dealing with particular ailments. By the 19th century in North America, if not elsewhere, they had been taken up by a variety of medical practitioners and entrepreneurs and were being collected and published for broader public distribution. A major part of this book has been the identification, compilation and selection of such home remedies.

A different but related development to these self-help remedies was the rapid growth in the latter part of the 19th century of the phenomenon of patent medicines. The reluctance of individuals to deal with the regular medical profession, combined with the entrepreneurial spirit of the time, encouraged the development of the patent medicine industry. The range of claims made by their proprietors was broad and often bizarre. Yet, they were attempting to satisfy individuals who felt that they wanted to, and indeed could, deal with their own ailments and treatments without the need of formal medical assistance.

Female midwifery was the third part of minority medicine during this period. Its status in communities in the birthing process, with women helping women, has not been fully recognized and credited. Midwives were of importance not only as caregivers, but also as knowledgeable keepers and translators of the self-help tradition.

The other division of minority medicine in 19th century Canada can be categorized as that of the practitioners of sectarian medicine. This diverse group can be defined as having or purporting to follow certain stated and broadly defined theoretical approaches to their particular view of medical treatment. They included the Thompsonians (Botanic medicine), Homeopathy, Eclecticism and the Entrepreneurs.

The story of Canada's social and economic development has been and can be told within a number of different frameworks, both temporal and geographic. Yet it is at the level of individuals and families, within their own time and place as they attempted to cope not only with daily common ailments, but often life-threatening illness, which concerns us here.

It was the substantial migration of individuals from Europe, particularly those from the British Isles, to North America which forms the background and the basis for this period. They included the Highland Scots to Cape Breton Island in the 1780s; the United Empire Loyalists into the remaining British colonies in North America in the 1780s; the Lowland Scots weavers to Lanark, Ontario; the Irish settlers brought by Peter Robinson to Peterborough, Ontario after the Napoleonic

Wars; the Irish famine emigrants in the 1840s; and the steady stream of immigrants throughout the remainder of the 19th century. And one cannot forget the settlement and development of the Canadian West which resulted from the movement not only of individuals from Ontario in the 1890s and beyond, but also from the substantial influx of varied ethnic groups from Europe and the United States.

It is almost impossible to give a complete cultural context or understanding for such a broad time period. It spans an era when it took eight weeks or more to cross the Atlantic on a sailing ship, to the arrival of steamships, and then to the transition from the horse and buggy to the iron rail and transcontinental travel. Yet, through time and with differing regional, social and cultural conditions, the spirit and purpose of the individuals involved remains a constant. These were individuals who faced hardship and sickness with a determination to deal with their own problems as best they could and with a belief in their obligation to help their neighbours.

The following anecdotal excerpts will perhaps give some context to, if not feeling for, this period:

> "Bad as it was on board, it became infinitely worse when we reached quarantine. On our arrival at the dock, ropes were stretched across the deck so as to leave a passage in the middle. A doctor was stationed on each side of this passage and only one person was allowed through at a time. All those who showed any symptoms of the disease [smallpox] were forced to go into quarantine, while others were sent ashore. The only exceptions made were in the cases of well mothers, who were permitted to accompany sick babes. I am an old man now, but not for a moment have I forgotten the scene as parents left children, brothers were parted from sisters, or wives and husbands were separated not knowing whether they should ever meet again. In some cases they never did meet again."
>
> *Report of Hugh Johnson, who left Glasgow, Scotland on June 18, 1847, for Quebec with his wife and two children, the youngest only three months old, in W. L. Smith,* The Pioneers of Old Ontario, *Toronto, 1923, pp. 208-209.*

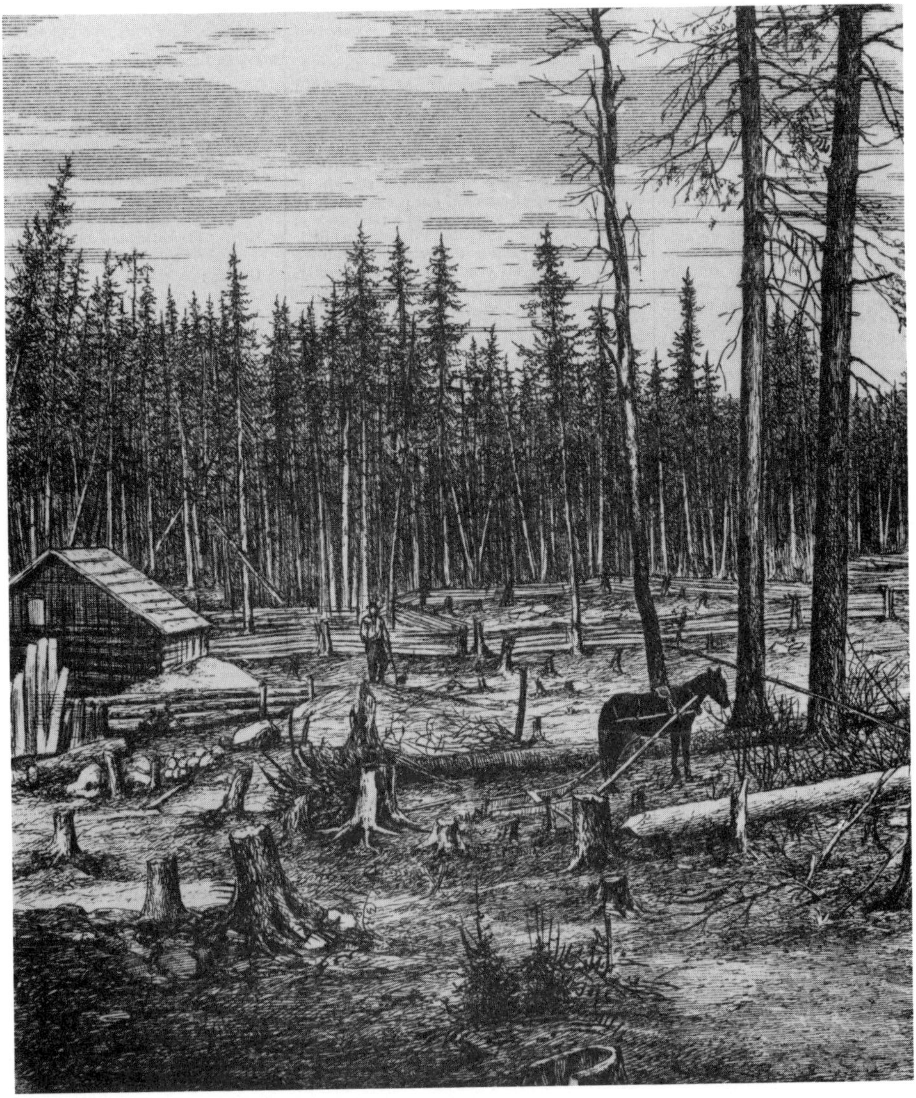

Forest clearing, *Canadian Illustrated News*, December 6, 1879

"The next day she appeared more lively but would not eat the arrowroot or sage which I prepared for her. She cried for bread, and of this we had none, not having been able to procure flour for some time for any money. It was a bitter trial, not having the thing for which she seemed to crave. The next day she fell into a stupor and about midnight the little angel spirit passed away to the immortal land. It pleased the Almighty to call our beloved child to Himself. Oh, gracious and almighty Father grant me thy grace to resign my darling infant to Thee. Thou gavest and Thou hast seen fit to take her. Oh God, thy will be done. Let not my turbulent heart rise, for Thou knowest best what is merciful. 'Ye have sorrowed now, but I will see you again and your heart shall rejoice and your joy no man taketh from you.' What comfort in these words."

The correspondence of Frances Stewart in October 1823, near Peterborough, Ont., commenting on her daughter Elizabeth's death from dysentery in Our Forest Home, being Extracts from the Correspondence of the late Frances Stewart, *Montreal, 1889, edited by E. S. Dunlop.*

❀❀❀

"For years, before doctors were available, men travelled miles to have wounds, which they had received in the bush, drawn together by a paste which father was skilled in making. Night after night, too, I have held a candle while he fashioned coffins for those who died."

Account of Mrs. John Shearer, Waterloo County, Ontario told in W. L. Smith, The Pioneers of Old Ontario, *Toronto, 1923, p. 203.*

❀❀❀

"A man named Gunn, who lived in Talbot Settlement, had rare skill in the setting of broken bones. He frequently travelled twenty-five miles on horseback over bush trails to set a broken limb."

Account from the north shore of Lake Erie, Ontario in the 1830s, in W. L. Smith, The Pioneers of Old Ontario, *Toronto, 1923, p. 224.*

"In this house there was a woman afflicted with acute rheumatism. She had tried the mineral oil without receiving any benefit from it, and consequently had been induced to put herself into the hands of one of the doctors of the settlement. This gentleman happened to make his daily visit when I was present, and entered the room, carrying a pair of large saddle-bags, in which phials and gallipots were heard clattering against each other in a most formidable manner. He did not deign to take off his hat, but advanced to his patient, and shook hands, saying, 'How d'ye do, my good lady, how d'ye do?'—'Oh, doctor,' cried the patient, 'I was wishing to see you—very bad—I don't calculate upon ever getting smart again.'—'Hoity, toity,' returned the doctor, 'you look a thundering sight better than you did yesterday.'—'Better!' exclaimed the sick woman, 'no, doctor, I am no better—I'm going to die in your hands.'—'My dear good lady,' cried the doctor, 'I'll bet a pint of spirits I'll raise you in five days, and make you so spry, that you'll dance upon this floor.'—'Oh,' said the woman, 'if I had but the root doctor that used to attend our family at Connecticut; he was a dreadful skeelful man.' Here they were interrupted by the entrance of her husband, who was a clumsy, credulous-looking person. 'Good morning to you, doctor,' said he, 'what's the word?'—'Nothing new or strange, sir,' returned the doctor. 'Well now, doctor,' continued the husband, 'how do you find that there woman?—no better, I conclude?—I guess as how it would be as well to let you understand plainly, that if you can't do her never no good, I wouldn't wish to be run into no expenses—pretty low times, doctor—money's out of the question. Now, sir, can you raise that there woman?'—'Yes, my good sir,' cried the doctor confidently, 'yes I can—I offered to bet a pint with her this moment, and I'll make it a quart if you please, my dear friend.'—'But, doctor, are you up to the natur (sic) of her ailment?' inquired the husband. 'Oh, perfectly,' said the other, 'nothing more simple; it arises entirely from obstruction and constitutional idiosyncrasy, and is seated under the muscular fascia. Some casual excitement has increased the action of the absorbent vessels so much, that they have drawn the blood from the different parts of the body, and occasioned the pain and debility that is now present.'—'Well now, doctor,' cried the husband, 'I swear you talk like a lawyer, and I begin to have hopes that you'll be pretty considerably apt to raise my woman.' The doctor now opened his saddlebags, and having set forth many small parcels and dirty phials upon the table, began to compound several recipes for his patient, who, when she saw him employed in this way, put our her head between the curtains of the bed, and cried, 'Doctor, don't forget to leave something for the debilitation.' When he had finished, he packed up his laboratory, and ordered that something he had left should be infused in a pint of whisky, and that a table-spoonful of the fluid should be taken three times a day.—'Will that raise me slick [soon]?' said the woman; 'I guess I had as well take it four times a day.' As the doctor was mounting his horse, I hear the farmer say, 'Doctor, don't be afeared about your pay, I'll see you satisfied; money, you know's, out of the question, but I've plenty of good buck-wheat."

Early account from southwestern Ontario in John Howison, Sketches of Upper Canada, *first published in 1821, Coles reprint, 1970, pp. 194-196.*

❀❀❀

"Few persons escape the second year without being afflicted with this weakening complaint [ague]; the mode of treatment is repeated doses of calomel, with castor-oil or salts, and is followed up by quinine. Those persons who do not choose to employ medical advice on the subject dose themselves with ginger-tea, strong infusion of Hyson, or any other powerful green tea; pepper, and whiskey; with many other remedies that have the sanction of custom or quackery."

Remarks of Catharine Parr Traill, near Rice Lake, Ontario, November 28, 1834, in Catharine Parr Traill, The Backwoods of Canada—Selections, *McClelland and Stewart, New Canadian Library, 1969, No. 5, p. 107.*

"This disease (dysentery) is often fatal to young children—frequently baffling the skill of the most experienced physician.

I lost two infants who were under the care of the most careful medical men; but saved another by the use of wild herb, that was given me by a Yankee settler's wife. A plant called spikenard (or spignet, as she called it), that grows in the forest, with a long spindle root, scraped, and a small quantity boiled in milk, thickens it, as if flour had been put in: it has a sweet astringent taste, slightly bitter. A tea-spoonful, thrice given in one day, cured the child, who was wasting fast under the disease. The spikenard belongs to the same family of plants, as the sarsaparilla: it bears black berries, not unlike the elderberry in size and taste. There are many of the old settlers who know the plant. No one should use the wild herbs without the experience of a careful person, to whom their sanatory or hurtful qualities are well known. The old Canadian settlers are often well skilled in the use of the native plants—they may, possibly, have learned the value of them from the Indians, or from long experience, taught by necessity, in a country where, formerly, educated doctors were far from being as commonly met with, even in the towns, as they now are. Possibly, in those days, there were fewer diseases to cure, and the simple medicines that the forest afforded were sufficient for all curative diseases. In lonely places, where the aid of a medical man is difficult to be obtained, even severe wounds are healed, and simple fractures are reduced by the inhabitants themselves. Some one among them who has more nerve, or more judgement than the rest, is consulted upon such occasions, and faith goes a great way with many patients in effecting a cure."

Remarks of Catharine Parr Traill near Rice Lake, Ontario, first published in 1855 in Catharine Parr Traill, The Canadian Settler's Guide, *Toronto, C.W., 1855, reprinted by McClelland and Stewart, New Canadian Library No. 64, 1969.*

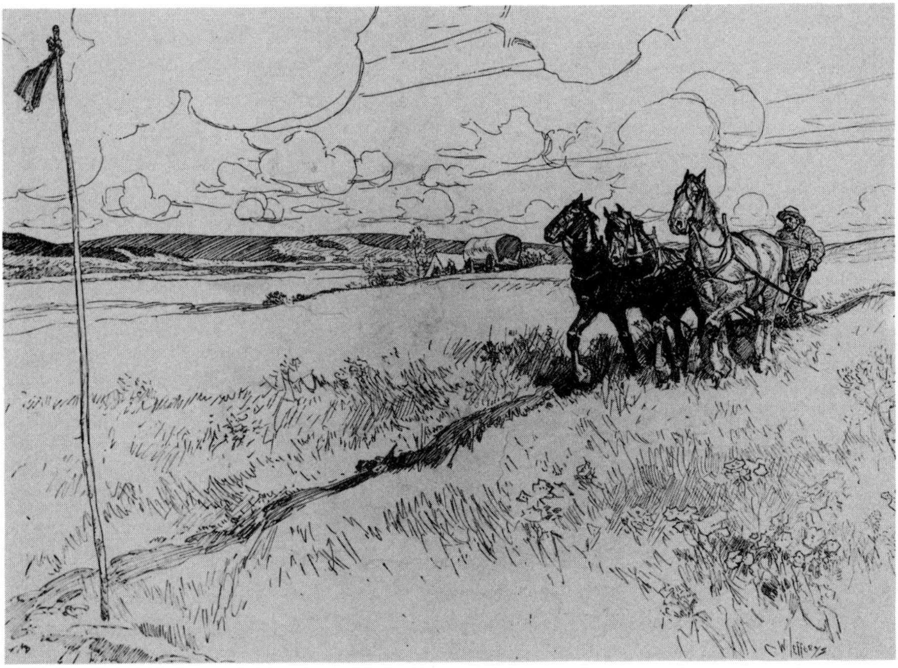

The First Furrow, C. W. Jefferys, National Archives of Canada, C73566, with permission of the C. W. Jefferys Estate Archives

"But the trials of that long first winter were not ended. In March the snow fell continually, it seemed, and with the wind shrieking over the plains, packing the snow in drifts as high as houses, we were entirely shut in. It was in this time of isolation that my eldest sister took sick, with a heavy cold, that in spite of turpentine and goose oil and mustard foot-baths, went steadily on through chills and fevers, until it seemed that she would die. She had reached a state of coma, her jaws were locked, and her eyes though still open, did not see. She lay, with her two long braids of bright brown hair, beside her little white face, a tired young traveller, ready to drop out of the race."

Comments of Nellie McClung, from rural Manitoba in the 1880s, Nellie L. McClung, Clearing in the West, *Toronto, Thomas Allen Ltd., 1935, p. 78.*

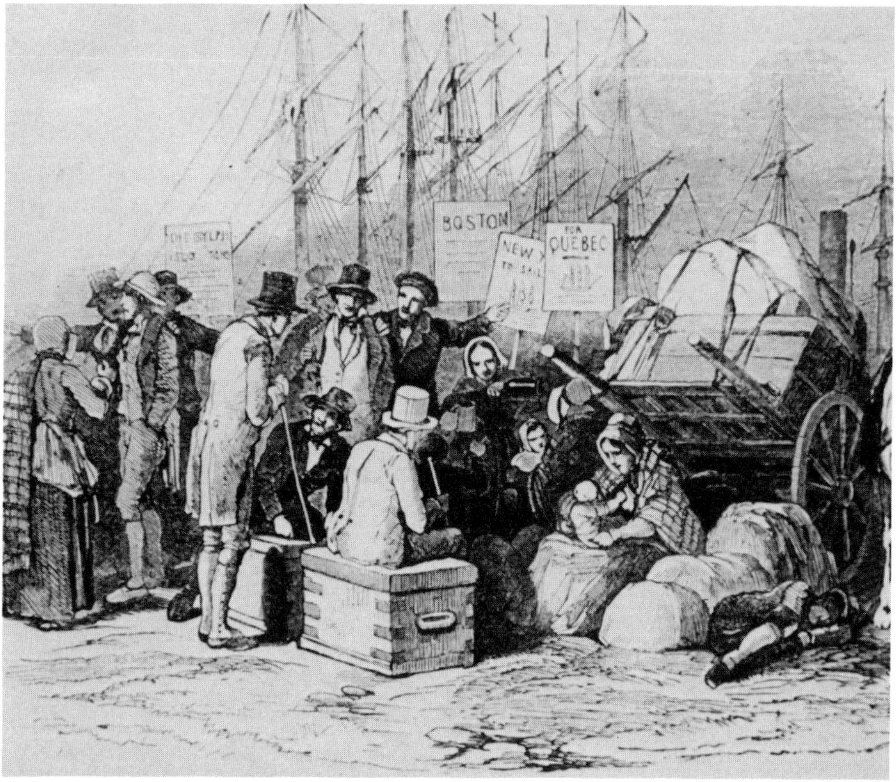

Irish Emigrants, *Illustrated London News*, May 10, 1851

What follows in this book is meant to give an overview, albeit a selective one, of self-help remedies as referred to and used in 19th century Canada. Several other aspects of minority medicine are briefly noted, as well as a variety of "sensible rules for good health" which were presented in self-help publications of the period. It is a time now gone, yet glimpses still remain. While some of the details may seem strange and unfamiliar, the essence of what follows still contains a message for the present.

Portraits from an Album

Faded grey photographs from the 19th century displayed in family albums or local histories, unrecognized and often unidentified—lost in the passage of time. Their faces and dress set a formal pose—somehow they are there, but not there—perhaps "a fragment of our collective character." Yet, they are the images of one's ancestors—although related by blood, they are known only from the brief references of an old favourite aunt. Lost because no one asked, lost because no one can remember. They were individuals we did not know; we did not speak to them or touch them. They were very real nevertheless, and coped with their own realities. Realities similar to our own—birth and death, love and hate, happiness and despair—in that sense, the normal human condition.

In the context of "good for what ails you" they dealt with their lives in ways so different from ours that we often have great difficulty relating to them. They were required to, and in many instances chose to, deal with their ailments on their own, whether by using self-help medicine with readily available ingredients or by relying on the myths of folk medicine. Unlike us, they could not banish sickness and death behind the sterile doors of institutional medicine. Sickness and death were an integral part of their homes and those who were caught unprepared suffered gravely. Women were responsible for the good health of their families, and the "receipts" found in this book were often their only resource in the days when medical training was rudimentary and professionally trained practitioners were few and far between.

The seven women featured in the accompanying photographs are representative of this tradition. Mother, daughters and granddaughters, who lived in Simcoe County, Ontario in the 19th century, they inherited and passed on their knowledge of "self-help remedies". Our generation's often instant rejection of this body of knowledge has quickly relegated it to the fading albums of memory. These portraits are meant to put a human face on what follows in this book—a human face with which one should never lose touch, whether in attempting to understand the past or in dealing with our present.

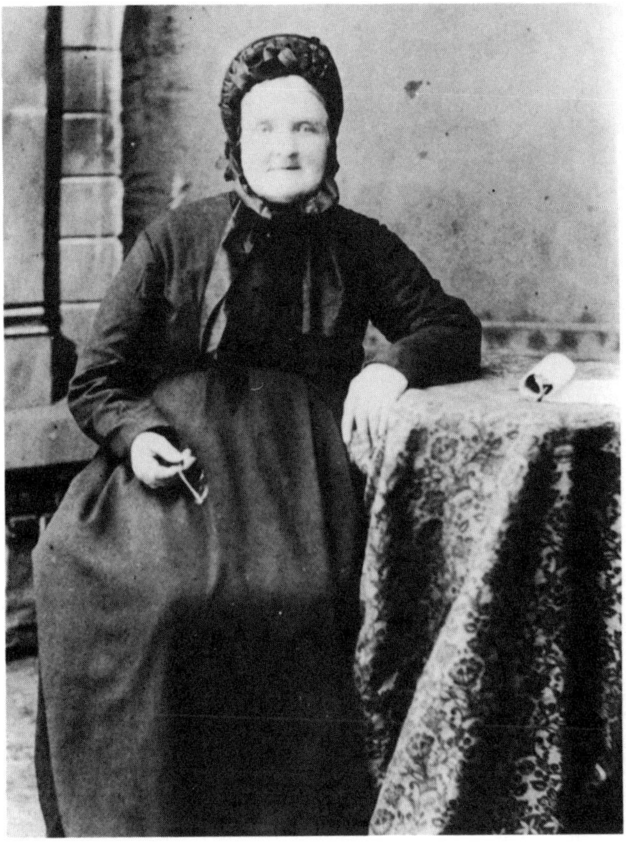

Mary Cameron Anderson

Born: Argyllshire, Scotland, 1824.

Died: June 17, 1900, Oro Township, Ontario.

Married: David Anderson (1820-1874), in Glasgow, Scotland, 1847.

Seven children were born in Scotland, two of whom (Ellen and David) died at age one, prior to the family emigrating to Canada in 1862. They settled on 100 acres (E 1/2 lot 9, Con. 14) in Oro Township, Simcoe County, Ontario, when the area was beginning to move beyond the frontier era. It was a time when people were born at home, died at home and were taken to the cemetery from their home. David and Mary are buried at Rugby, Ontario.

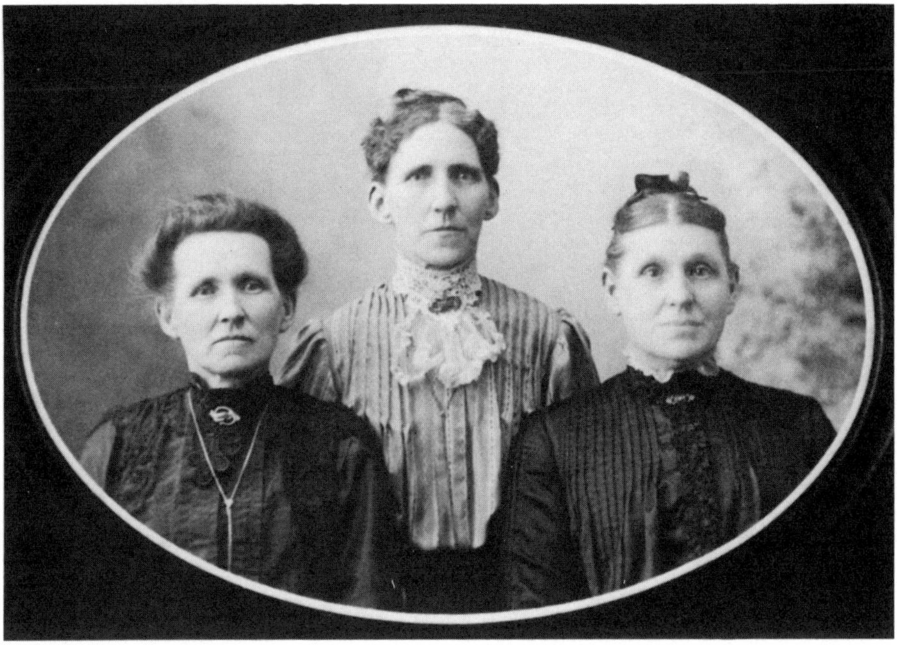

The Three Daughters of Mary Cameron Anderson

	Helen (Ellen)	Catherine (Katie)	Mary
Born:	1856	1862	1853-1930
Married:	John Smith	Noah Payne	Robert Miller Roberts

Mary Anderson was born in Glasgow, Scotland, on January 9, 1853 and emigrated at the age of nine with her family to Oro Township. On November 21, 1873, she married Robert Miller Roberts (1842-1928), whose first wife had died during childbirth in 1871. The Roberts family (weavers) had emigrated from Glasgow in 1843/44 to Oro and took up land which backed on to the Anderson property. Mary and Robert had nine children (three girls and six boys) all of whom grew up on the family farm (W 1/2 lots 8 and 9, Con 14). Mary Anderson Roberts died at her home on September 5, 1930.

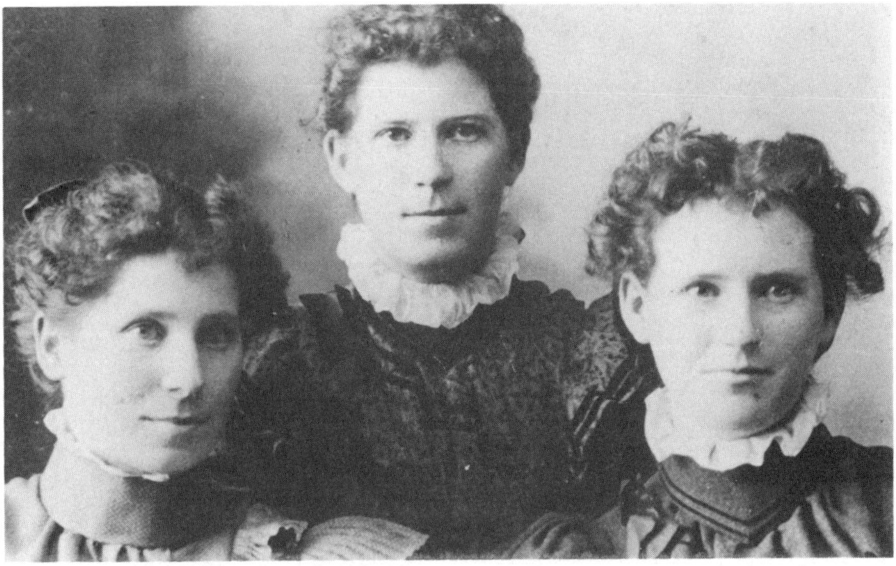

The Three Daughters of Mary Anderson Roberts

	Mary Cameron	Catherine Ellen (Nell)	Marion Miller (Little Minnie)
Born:	1874-1938	1879-1971	1878-1965
Married:	J.A.R. Cameron	Robert Marshall	

Mary Cameron Roberts, the oldest child of Mary and Robert Roberts, was born on November 24, 1874 on their farm. She married James Alexander Robertson Cameron (1872-1933), on March 28, 1906 in Oro. Mary's future husband had travelled in 1899 with one of her younger brothers (Andrew Nelson Roberts) to look for new opportunities in the Canadian West. On July 6, 1899, J.A.R. Cameron took entry upon a quarter section of land as a homestead patent for the NE 1/4 of Section 14, Township 10, Range 17a of the 2nd Meridian in the North West Territories, near the community of Yellow Grass in the soon-to-become (1905) Province of Saskatchewan. By 1905, he had broken and cropped 36 acres and had four oxen, one cow, a 12x16 ft. house worth $50, and a stable worth $50. In 1906, he returned to Oro where he married Mary Roberts. They went west and remained on their farm near Yellow Grass from 1906 to 1922, where their three children were all born at home. Following their return to Ontario, they lived in Barrie until their deaths in the 1930s.

Look For The Lilacs

I met an old man walking on the gravel road,
We stopped, I idly, he to rest his load
Of berries in a rusty pail,
Blueberries, and he offered some for sale,
And I a cigarette. We sat then on a sun warmed rock,
Ate berries, rested, had a little talk
Of weather, bears and politics and means and ways,
And so he came to speak of boyhood days.
Turn of the century and some before,
Not much here then, one hotel, a store,
A blacksmith shop, a mill to grind the grain
From hard-won farms, the lumber trade, the train,
Although the station twenty miles away,
The stage over the rocky ridges, mineral, marsh hay
To see the beasts through winter, and my wonder grew
To hear of all the farms, so many, I had thought so few.
"Why now, look for the lilacs", that is what he said
And rose and pointed to the hills ahead,
"Grown now to popple mostly and to pine,
But that was farms back in my father's time.
Each to his grant along the settlers road
Cut pine, built his log cabin and then sowed
What seed he brought between the stumps that year
To get what crop he could. There was the fear,
you see, of hunger. But they wintered through
Though some had lost their woman or a child or two.
Speaking of that, my grandad used to say
It took three wives to raise a family in his day,
But, just like women, just as soon as ever
They saw their brood roofed in against the weather,
The chimney built, root cellar dug, a garden plot,
They turned their minds to flowers, and they got
Cuttings from out front, lilacs and roses and the rest,
Of all it was the lilacs did the best,
Took to the soil. Well, well, all gone and past,
The land wore out, the pine was done at last,
Folks moved away, clearings went back to woods,
The roofs fell in and where the cabins stood
Is just the cellar holes. But you will know
Each place,
Come May, you'll mark the lilacs blow.

Look for the Lilacs, *Barbara Lester, Cloyne, Ontario, 1984.*

Good For What Ails You

> A person may live long, however, and yet be a sufferer from either occasional or continuous ills, which may be hard to bear, without being necessarily fatal; and the farmer himself may be in good health, and yet be much troubled and put to an expense through troubles within the family circle, among those who labour in the household.
>
> *The Canada Farmer,* November 15, 1876.

One capsule three times daily before meals. It's written on that little slip of paper with the indecipherable chemical symbols, and the even less-easily deciphered signature of the prescribing medical professional. We take it to the local drugstore, crossing our fingers that the pharmacist can make more sense out of the scrawl than we, the potential ingestors of that capsule. Unlike the prescriptions of today, the following receipts/recipes/remedies contained no secret codes and it did not take a trained pharmacologist to understand them. They are not meant to be or seen to be merely "a hodgepodge of concoctions," but rather the author's selective compilation of remedies which were recommended and used during the period.

What is the social context in which these remedies should be set? My adoptive maternal grandmother, Helen Ross McIntyre, whom I knew very well, was born in 1878. Indeed, 19th century Canada, in a temporal sense, has only recently passed. Yet it is by today's standards almost another world. Much, if not most, of Canada was rural and small community based. The context of health care was focused on the family's self-reliance, prior to the medical infrastructure and the modern scientific models which we have come to accept today. As an important aside, let me note that the significant medical advances which have occurred since this period have significantly enhanced not only our life spans, but also our quality of life. Having said that, it must be noted that such change also has led to an institutionalization of health care systems and an often related loss of personal responsibility for one's own health.

What are the sources of the following home remedies? The answer is that they are many and varied. Unfortunately, it is very difficult to identify in given families or communities across Canada which particular remedies were used when, where, and how often. As in all commentaries on social history, it is impossible to know with certainty how the past was constructed and operated. Yet, through the identification and interpretation of published materials of the time, one can attempt to reconstruct a partial context.

During this period, a large number of "self-help" publications were produced, some perhaps with humanitarian aims, others for commercial purposes. Yet, they all had recognized the public need if not demand for the information which they contained. Or, as illustrated and poignantly noted in the title of Mary Morris' thirty-five page work (London, 1764), *Every one their own PHYSICIAN: or, CHARITY made pleasant, by relieving their own FAMILY, or poor neighbouring PEOPLE, by cheap, easy and safe REMEDIES.* Let us look for a moment at some of these publications.

Dr. Alvin Wood Chase (1817-1885) was born in Cayuga County, New York, and died in Ann Arbor, Michigan. Having received his medical training in the eclectic tradition, and having perceived a need if not a market, he produced several books for popular consumption. *Dr. Chase's Recipes or Information for Everybody* by A.W. Chase, M.D., practical therapeutist, Ann Arbor, Michigan, had reached its twelfth edition by 1863. *Dr. Chase's Family Physician, Bee-Keeper and Second Receipt Book* appeared in 1873 with several Canadian editions (London, Ontario, 7th Canadian, 1882). A final book appeared after his death—*Dr. Chase's Third, Last and Complete Receipt Book and Household Physician or Practical Knowledge for the People*, F. B. Dickerson Co.; Detroit and Windsor, 1890.

Dr. Chase's receipt books contain a large and varied range of material. Their medical sections provide symptoms and treatments for a variety of illnesses and ailments. The remedies and his remarks are generally very detailed and often include his sources and the names of individuals who had benefited from their use. Sections on nursing, midwifery and cooking, both for the sick and the healthy, are included. In addition, sections deal with household miscellanea, the toilet, domestic and farm animals and even machines. The dedication to the 1887 book notes that "twelve hundred thousand families" throughout the United States and Canada had purchased one or both of his previous books. Clearly his efforts had struck a responsive chord, as Dr. Chase notes with some stridency, yet humility, in 1863:

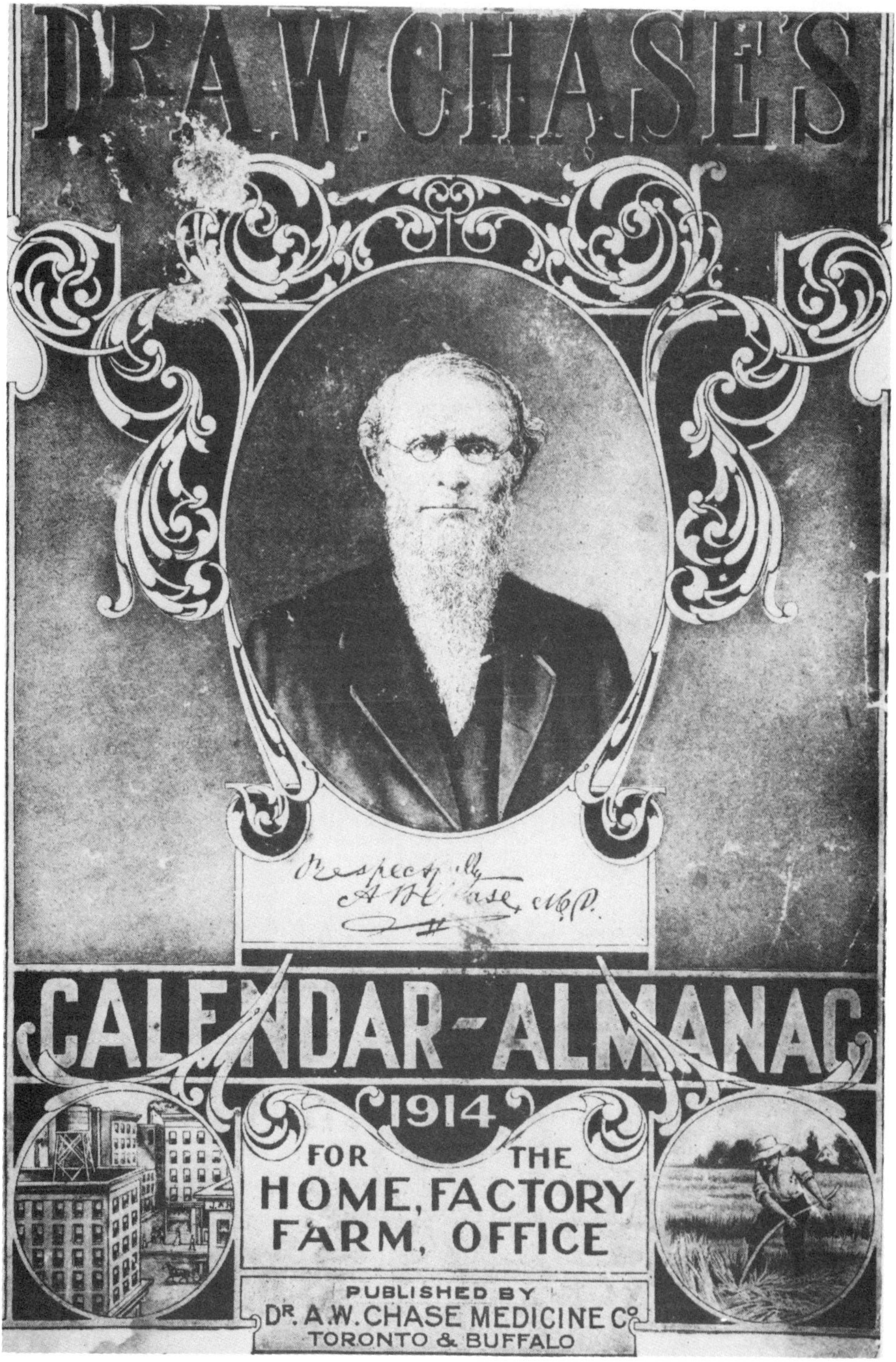

City of Vaughan Archives

> Many persons will stick up their noses at these "Old Grandmother prescriptions," but I tell many "upstart Physicians" that our grandmothers are carrying more information out of the world by their deaths, than will ever be possessed by this class of "sniffers," and I really thank God, as do thousands of others, that He has enabled me, in this work, to reclaim such an amount of it for the benefit of the world.

The Household Guide or Domestic Cyclopedia - Home Remedies for Man and Beast (J. L. Nichols, Toronto, 1894, 14th edition) is also typical of this genre. By 1899, it had gone to its 20th edition. It claims to provide "a practical home physician, home remedies and home treatment for all diseases" and "an instructor on nursing, housekeeping and home adornments." In addition, it contains "a complete cook book" by Mrs. J. L. Nichols. The book is well illustrated with line drawings and its 1899 edition of 539 pages contains subheadings such as health, disease, home remedies and how to use them, sick-room hints, care and feeding of infants, the hygiene of the bedroom and a complete medical dictionary.

The People's Home Library: A Library of Three Practical Books appeared in a number of editions (1916, 1917, 1920) published by R. C. Barnum, Cleveland and Imperial Publishing, Toronto. Its 1044 pages contain three main separate sections—a home medical book, a home recipe book and a home stock [animal] book. The medical section contains hundreds of practical self-help remedies organized under parts of the body and their particular ailments.

A large number of other self-help books were available throughout this period. The following excerpts provide a perspective:

> Health is certainly more valuable than money, because it is by health that money is produced; but thousands and millions are of small avail, to alleviate the protracted tortures of the gout, to repair the broken organs of sense, or resuscitate the powers of digestion.
>
> Poverty is, indeed, an evil from which we naturally fly; but let us not run from one enemy to another, nor take shelter in the arms of sickness.
>
> *Family Receipts: or Practical Guide for the Husbandman and Housewife*, H. L. Barnum, Cincinnati, 1831.

THE

HOUSEHOLD GUIDE

OR

DOMESTIC CYCLOPEDIA.

HOME REMEDIES FOR MAN AND BEAST;

A COMPLETE RECEIPT BOOK.

Home Nursing and Home Treatment;

Insect Extermination;

PROF. HENKEL'S ILLUSTRATIONS OF THE EFFECTS OF ALCOHOL & CIGARETTES;

CARE OF CHILDREN;

HOW TO COOK FOR THE SICK, Etc.

—BY—

PROF. B. G. JEFFERIS, M. D., Ph. D., Chicago, Ill.,

AND

J. L. NICHOLS, A. M.

ALSO,

A COMPLETE COOK BOOK,

—BY—

Mrs. J. L. NICHOLS.

FOURTEENTH EDITION.

PUBLISHED BY

J. L. NICHOLS & CO.,

No. 33 Richmond St. West,

TORONTO, ONTARIO,

To whom all communications must be addressed.

1894.

In preparing a new work as a "guide to health," I have been influenced mainly by the conviction that such a work was very much required. Having travelled considerably during the last two years, and mixed much with the agricultural population, I have been concerned to see that in a large proportion of cases, the health of the inhabitants was not what it should be. Some of this deficiency may doubtless be ascribed to the vicissitudes of climate; some to hardships necessarily attendant on the labours and privations of first-settlers; but still more to a careless neglect of those "rules of health," attention to pure air, cleanliness, exercise and food, that are absolutely necessary if we would enjoy life. Some of this arises from ignorance, some from carelessness, and some from stinginess. Many men will allow disease to accumulate in their families for months, depending occasionally upon quack medicines, rather than send for a medical man. In many cases the medical man does not live conveniently, and they grudge the expense of the visits.

Smith's Family Physician, Toronto, Hunter, Rose & Co., 1869

❀❀❀

Believing in the sound principle that "an ounce of prevention is worth a pound of cure," the publishers confidently present this volume to the public, in the hope it will fill a long felt want in the community.

The purpose of the work is to fully inform every man and woman what are the real causes of sickness and what are the most approved methods of treatment. And moreover it is especially intended as an aid to home or domestic treatment in the thousand cases where a physician cannot readily be reached, and when, if ordinary common sense is used, his services are not required.

The Family Physician or Everyman His Own Doctor, compiled by leading Canadian medical men, Toronto, Rose Publishing Co., 1889.

What, then, can be presented as an overview or theme among the following self-help remedies? The approaches were all common sense and practical. The ingredients were readily available, whether salt, onions or garden herbs. The numerous historical sources for such remedies all provide, not unexpectedly, a similar range and focus. Colds and coughs were most often noted, followed by rheumatism/arthritis; stomach complaints (diarrhoea/constipation/indigestion); and the skin (warts/burns). Salves and poultices for a wide range of ailments were also commonly noted.

Clearly most of these ailments were not life-threatening—yet they had to be coped with, if not cured, within the social and medical context of the period. And indeed they were. Perhaps an appropriate way to conclude this introduction to home remedies is to refer to the commentary in The *Canada Farmer* of 1868 (Vol. 5, p. 79) which noted that one of the Ten Follies was "to advise another to take a remedy which you have tried yourself without making special inquiry whether all the conditions are alike."

Infectious Diseases

Diphtheria

A gargle composed of vinegar, honey and warm water is an excellent remedy. For adults add red pepper.

❀

Have the patient inhale the steam from lime water.

❀

Insert a funnel over some pitch tar on a hot iron and let the patient breathe the smoke five or six times a day. Also let the patient hold small pieces of ice in the mouth.

❀

Gargle with salt and water and apply bandages wet with salt and water to the throat and bind on slices of fat bacon.

❀

Take a common tobacco pipe; place a live coal in the bowl; drop a little tar upon the coal. Draw the smoke into the mouth and discharge it through the nostrils. When the smoke is drawn into the mouth it will irritate the throat and cause a spasm of coughing, which in some cases, dislodged the membrane that formed in the throat as the result of the infection.

Influenza (grippe)

For sore throat and cough use the following: vinegar, 1 teacupful; honey, 1/2 teacupful; cayenne, 1 teaspoonful; simmer together for a few minutes and when cool give a teaspoonful whenever the cough is troublesome.

❀

Live on a pure milk diet for several days. If milk does not agree add a large tablespoonful of lime water for each teacupful. Boil the milk before giving it to the patient and let him sip it with a teaspoon, instead of drinking it.

❀

Put the patient to bed and surround him with hot bricks or irons until the sweat pours from him. Keep the patient in bed until all moisture is gone and stay in a warm room until well. Allow plenty of fresh air but avoid sitting where the breeze will strike you.

If the case is severe the patient should go to bed and hot water bottles should be placed at the sides and feet. Also drink pennyroyal, peppermint or sage tea.

Lock Jaw (tetanus)

Moisten some tobacco thoroughly and lay upon the patient's stomach. This will cause sickness and relaxing of the muscles as there are many nerves in this region. Do not leave it on longer than is necessary to produce the desired effect or it may cause deathly sickness.

❀

Put hot wood ashes into hot water, wet thick cloths in the water and apply to the jaws as quickly as possible and at the same time bathe the entire backbone with hot vinegar with either cayenne pepper or mustard added. If vinegar is not at hand use hot water in its place. Persist in this treatment and the jaws will relax.

❀

Let anyone who has an attack of lock jaw take a small quantity of spirits of turpentine; warm it and pour it into the wound—no matter what the wound is, or what its nature is—and relief will follow in less than one minute.

Measles

To relieve the itching, frequently bathe the patient with warm, weak lye water.

❀

A mild and safe way to treat measles is to sponge off frequently the entire body, changing the clothes at each bath. Avoid draughts, yet have the room well ventilated. Drink freely of pure water, cold or hot tea, as the patient relishes. Keep the bowels loose, and have the diet cooling and nutritious. If the eyes are affected darken the room, lay over them cool cloths and bathe to allay nervousness.

❀

If there is any diarrhoea give blackberry root tea.

❀

If there is inflammation of the lungs apply a mustard poultice to the chest and follow with a poultice of hops and lobelia. Change every half hour.

Scarlet Fever

Take cayenne pepper, 1 teaspoonful; common salt, 2 teaspoonfuls and a teacupful of water with enough vinegar added to make of the desired strength. Bring these to the boiling point, let stand until cool and then strain. Use as a gargle for sore throat either in colds or scarlet fever.

❀

The sick person should be kept in a room apart from the rest of the family. The room should be kept at a temperature of 65 degrees, light a fire if possible, and leave the windows down at the top. Admit fresh air freely; if cold weather cover the patient's head and body well. Give a bath daily (of course under the approval of the physician), rub dry quickly. Keep the feet and legs warm, and guard against a check in perspiration. Notice the breathing at night to see if there be trouble with the air passages. See if the limbs swell, and report all changes to the physician. The skin becomes dry and begins to scale off the fifth or sixth day after the rash appears. No patient should be allowed to leave the bed until this process is complete. The warm baths should be kept up, chillness guarded against and the room kept at about 70. After recovery the patient should be kept in the room two weeks, and when allowed to go out should be well wrapped up.

The troubles that may arise from carelessness often result fatally in dropsy, sore throat, disease of the kidneys, and other malignant maladies which follow scarlet fever, and too much care cannot be taken.

❀

Cut an onion in half; take out the heart; put a spoonful of saffron into the cavity; put the pieces together again; wrap in a cloth and bake in an oven. When the onion is cooked so that the juice will run freely, squeeze out all the juice and give a teaspoonful to the patient. Rub goose grease or a piece of bacon on the chest and throat. Keep the patient warm and seldom any other treatment will be required. The saffron keeps the bowels open and the onion is soothing to the sore and congested throat.

❀

For vomiting, give the patient small chips of ice in the mouth.

❀

An eminent physician says that if he were confined to one single remedy in cases of scarlet fever, he should choose lard. Rub the little sufferer with it thoroughly and often. It allays the fever and softens the parched skin. The amount thus absorbed is simply astonishing.

Keep the patient in bed and give a fluid diet of milk gruel, beef tea, etc., with plenty of cold water to drink. Control the fever by sponging the body with tepid water, and relieve the pain in the throat by cold compresses, applied externally. As soon as the skin shows a tendency to become scaly, apply goose grease or clean lard with a little boracic acid powder dusted in it, or better, perhaps, carbolized vaseline, to relieve the itching and prevent the scales from being scattered about and subjecting others to the contagion.

Whooping Cough

Mix equal parts of licorice, sulphur, fresh butter and spermaceti. This may be taken freely.

❀

The tincture made of the fresh root of skunk cabbage is good for whooping cough. The dose is from 1 to 2 drams.

❀

Make a tea of peach leaves by adding an ounce of the leaves to a pint of cold water and allowing to stand until the water has taken part of their strength. Give a tablespoonful every hour or two.

❀

The inhalation of air charged with ammonia vapours, as a remedy for whooping cough, has been tried with success. One of the methods of application employed is boiling strong ammonia in the room where the patient is.

❀

Take a good handful of sunflower seed. Steep in 1 cup of water for an hour and take 1 pint of sumach bobs and steep in 2 cups of water for an hour. Mix the 3 cups of juice together, sweeten with honey, let the patient take a sip of this every time he whoops. It soon checks the whoop. It is also splendid for the flu.

❀

For whooping cough put one cupful of saltpetre in a saucepan with half a cupful of water. Let it stand on the side of the stove until the saltpetre is melted, then take some thick white blotting paper and cut it into four-inch squares and soak them in the saltpetre. Dry them in the sun, and burn one square in the bedroom at night on a tin or enamel or china plate. This is also a very good cure for ordinary colds.

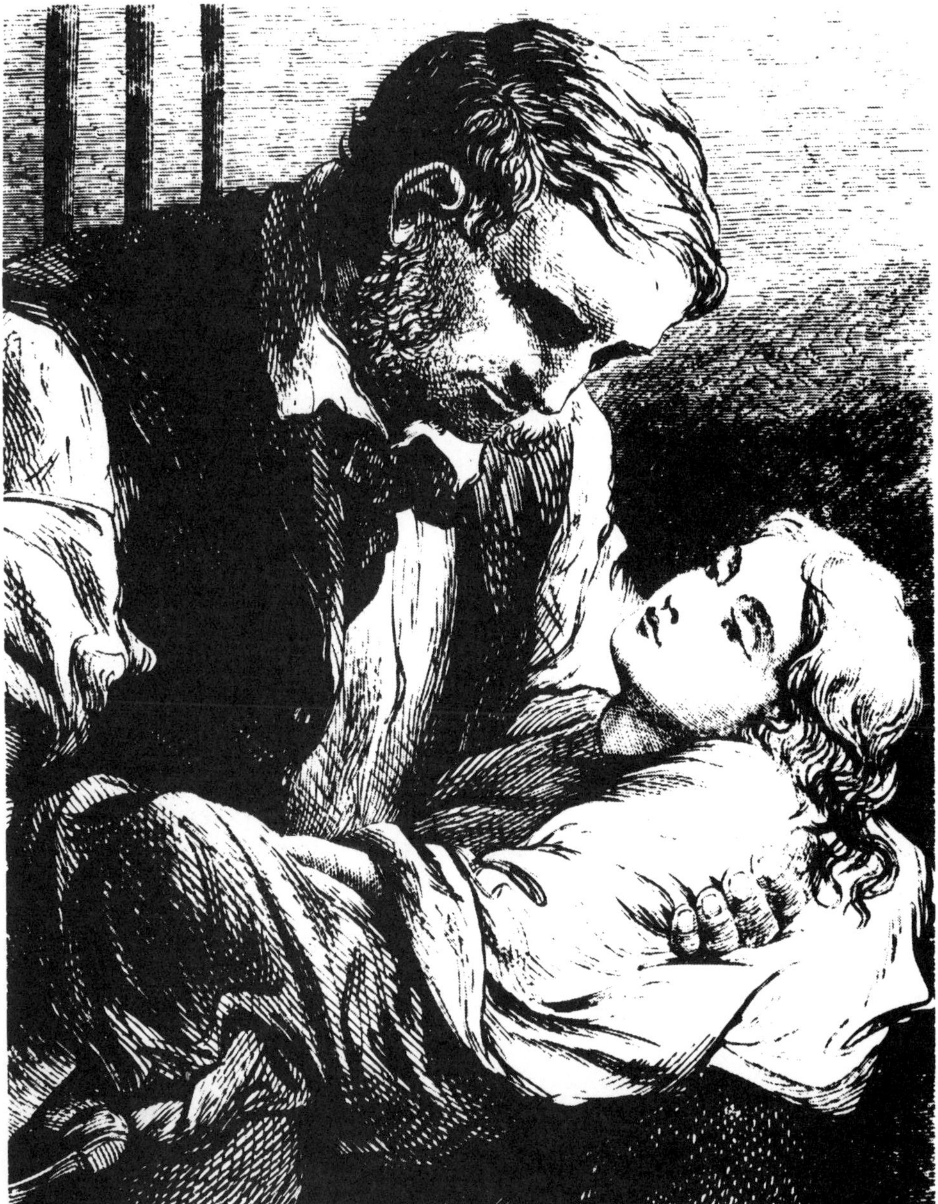

Boil some pine boughs, wintergreen and sweet oil and use the solution.

❀

Flaxseed tea taken frequently is excellent for whooping cough. A fresh egg dropped in lemon juice, and let dissolve will also give relief.

❀

For an effective syrup take sliced onions and garlics, of each 1 gill; sweet oil 1 gill; stew them in the oil, in a covered dish, to obtain the juices; then strain and add honey 1 gill; paregoric and spirits of camphor, of each 1/2 oz.; bottle and cork tight for use. Dose for a child of 2 or 3 years, 1 teaspoon 3 or 4 times daily, or whenever the cough is troublesome, increasing or decreasing, according to age.

❀

Patient should eat plain food and avoid cold drafts and damp air, but keep in the open air as much as possible. A strong tea made of the tops of red clover is highly recommended. A strong tea made of chestnut leaves, sweetened with sugar, is also very good.

❀

Seven large carrots, 5 medium turnips and 2 large onions. Do not peel the carrots or turnips. Scrub with brush until clean. Grind them all to a pulp or grate finely. Squeeze out all the juice and save. Put 1 pound of Rock Candy and 1 quart of water in a clean saucepan and boil slowly until 1 pint remains. Strain, let cool and give 1/2 to 1 teaspoonful every hour until relief comes.

Intestinal Disorders

Colic

Give babies plenty of warm water that has been boiled and always use a bottle with a nipple.

❀

Put a mustard plaster over the pain and if the bowels are constipated give an injection of salt and molasses, castor oil, or soap and warm water.

❀

Injections of salt and water will almost always give instant relief from colic.

❀

A good remedy is nothing more nor less than glycerine, as much as the child will take. It is best to begin with a teaspoonful, but there is no fear of giving too much. The first effect is the quieting of the cry of pain; the second, the belching of the gas; later the gas passes away downward, and finally, after an easy movement of the bowels, the child falls into a sweet, restful sleep. Try it, its efficacy will surprise you, as will also the readiness with which the little one will suck it from the spoon.

❀

Pour hot water upon a little soot from the chimney and have the child drink it. It seems to absorb all the gas.

❀

Vinegar weakened with water and taken as a drink is a good remedy for many cases of colic.

❀

For cramp colic give a wineglassful of olive oil. For cramps, rubbing the parts thoroughly with the hands or a piece of flannel will generally produce relief. The application of turpentine or spirits of hartshorn, rubbed on with the hand, is highly recommended.

❀

For flatulent or common wind colic give, as an emetic, either a teaspoonful of mustard or salt to a teacupful of water. This may be repeated in 10 or 12 minutes if necessary. This is for colic caused by food in the stomach.

The white of an egg, warm water, brandy and nutmeg, a wineglassfull is good for the colic.

❀

If there is constipation with the colic give an injection of an ounce of warm peppermint tea with a teaspoonful of castor oil in it. Spearmint tea will do in place of peppermint.

❀

Give the baby some onion tea if it has the colic. This is also good for a fretful baby and is not injurious like many of the soothing syrups which are used.

❀

For an infant's syrup use 1 lb. best box raisins; 1/2 ounce of anise seed; two sticks licorice; split the raisins, pound the anise seed, and cut the licorice fine; add to it 3 quarts of rain water, and boil down to 2 quarts. Feed three or four times a day, as much as the child will willingly drink. The raisins strengthen, the anise expels the wind, and the licorice is a physic.

❀

A few tablespoonfuls of hot water will often allay a severe attack of the colic. Catnip tea is also a good remedy.

❀

A drop of essence of peppermint in 6 or 7 teaspoonfuls of hot water will give relief.

Constipation

For constipation eat plenty of rhubarb.

❀

Mix charcoal with a little molasses and take from a teaspoonful to a tablespoonful as often as required to produce the desired effects. At the same time it will be well to bathe the bowels occasionally with vinegar to which a little pepper has been added. The molasses is loosening and the charcoal is an antiseptic.

❀

Bean biscuit is good for constipation. To prepare this take 1 pint of beans, 1/2 pint of flour, 4 teaspoonfuls of molasses or sugar, sour milk with soda to sweeten, and a piece of butter the size of an egg. Make quite a thick batter and bake in gem pans. Eat two biscuits at each meal until relieved.

❀

Women of sedentary habits are often troubled with costiveness, to prevent which use a little rhubarb occasionally; either chew it or take a small portion in hot water sweetened; accustom yourself to use Indian Meal, or unbolted wheat meal made into bread; this course has cured thousands.

❀

One-half pound of good figs chopped fine, one-half pint of molasses, two ounces powdered senna leaves, one dram fine powdered coriander seed, one dram of fine powdered cardamom seed. Put the molasses on the stove and let it come to a boil, then stir in all the rest and bring to a boil again. A teaspoonful once in a while is a dose. It will keep, when covered, for a year.

❀

Squeeze the juice from a half a lemon and add about 3 tablespoonfuls of water and a teaspoonful of sugar and drink before breakfast every morning for a week or ten days. This is very good.

❀

A tablespoon of corn meal stirred up in sufficient cold water and drunk in the morning, immediately after rising, has, with perseverance, cured many bad cases.

❀

In old age, a daily drive or gentle massage of the bowels are often advisable. Horseback exercise will benefit a good many. Some cases, where constipation is due to a nervous or dynamic cause, yield to high grade homeopathy. More fats, such as butter, in the dietary help others. But however hard the problem may be, more study is what is called for, not a laxative medicine.

❀

Constipation may be relieved by mixing two ounces of senna boiled in a quart of water with one pound of stewed prunes and half a teacup of sugar; take a tablespoonful of the mixture before each meal. Ripe fruit before breakfast and dried fruit freely eaten at meals are simple and effective remedies.

Let no remedy, however, divert attention from the great abuse, an abuse from which constipation must be expected and considered due—that of swallowing food without masticating it well.

❀

When nature calls, at either door, do not attempt to bluff-her;
But haste-away, night or day, or health is sure to suffer.

The above with attention to diet, using milk, roasted apples, and if not dyspeptic, uncooked apples, pears, peaches, etc. at meal time, "Yankee Brown Bread," or bread made of unbolted wheat, if preferred, and avoiding a meat diet, will in most cases soon remedy the difficulty.

❀

A cup of hot water is a grand tonic and stomach cleanser, and a sure cure for constipation. It should be taken night and morning, just before retiring and after rising.

❀

Beware of harsh purgatives, they make matters worse. A regular hour each day must be established for going to stool. Sufficient time must be taken to permit the bowels to become thoroughly evacuated. Careful regulation of the diet; not too much nor too little food should be taken. Avoid tea, cheese, crackers, all highly seasoned food, and eat plenty of fruit with coarse bread, such as graham and cornmeal, gingerbread made with molasses, and oatmeal porridge. Plenty of water should be taken between meals. These rules should be rigidly enforced before any permanent cure can be hoped for.

❀

Two simple procedures will usually restore normal action to the bowels. Drink a pint of cold water before breakfast, a half a spoonful or less at a time, that is, in little sips, the whole sipping exercise taking at least twenty minutes. Chew the food to a cream; so thoroughly, that is, that it can not very well go into solid form again, but will blend with the digestive juices, particularly the bile, and remain fluid.

❀

If the child is nursed regularly and held out at the same time of each day, it will seldom be troubled with this complaint. Give plenty of water. Regularity of habit is the best remedy. If this method fails, use a soap suppository. Make it by paring a piece of white castile soap round. It should be made about the size of a lead pencil, pointed at the end.

Cream and butter are to be recommended on porridge and cornmeal. Oatmeal gruels should be used by older children, who should also be encouraged to drink as much water as they crave. For children three years and older, stewed prunes, orange juice, honey and bread, olive oil and olives, peaches, fresh vegetables and baked apples and gingerbread should form part of the bill of fare, and there will be no need of castor oil, rhubarb, etc., often an injury to the child.

Diarrhoea and Summer Complaints

Melted sheep's tallow is fine for this trouble. Give 2 tablespoonfuls every 2 hours.

❀

Take and tie a pint of flour very tightly in a cloth and put into boiling water. When untied the gluten of the flour will be found outside on the ball, remove this and the inside will prove a dry powder which is very astringent. Grate this and wet a portion of it in cold milk. Boil a pint of milk and when it is at the boiling point stir in as much of the wet mixture as will thicken it to the quality of palatable porridge. Stir in a little salt and let this be the sole article of diet until the disease has disappeared. Relieve it first by toasted bread or very delicate mutton broth which latter is also astringent if the disease has not progressed to the degree of inflammation. This diet will generally preclude the use of medicine.

❀

The common mullein leaf boiled in new milk, and sweetened, is a very effective remedy for all complaints of the bowels.

❀

A strong solution of common baking soda is an excellent remedy for diarrhoea.

❀

Burn some pulverized rhubarb to black ashes in an iron dish, then powder it and give half a teaspoonful three times a day in a little water. Rhubarb will discharge all irritating material and burning it makes it somewhat antiseptic.

❀

Chronic diarrhoea is frequently cured by drinking tea made of orange peel, sweetened with loaf sugar, and drank freely, for six or seven days.

Stir lightly into a teacup of cold water the white of one egg not beaten. This forms a coating on the stomach, and is very nourishing. Slippery elm gruel is another simple remedy. A tablespoonful of flour stirred in a glass of water, sometimes checks the disease promptly. Ice water enemas after each action of the bowels is sometimes beneficial.

❀

Slice some smoked fat bacon and fry it until you have half a pint of grease. While it is frying, slice several large onions into the grease and when it is done pour off the mixture. The dose is a teaspoonful once a day.

❀

Drink freely of hot milk. The milk should not be boiled but should be heated as hot as it can be drunk.

❀

Apply an onion poultice to the bowels or a cloth wrung out of turpentine.

❀

Take Indian corn, roasted and ground in the manner of coffee, or coarse meal browned, and boil in a sufficient quantity of water to produce a strong liquid, like coffee, and drink a teacupful warm, two or three times a day. One day's practice, it is said, will ordinarily effect a cure.

❀

Blackberry cordial is said to be almost a specific for summer complaint or diarrhoea. From a teaspoonful to a wineglass is to be taken, according to the age of the patient, until relieved. Following is a recipe for making blackberry cordial: To two quarts of juice add one pound of white sugar; half ounce nutmeg, half ounce cinnamon, pulverized; half ounce cloves, pulverized. Boil all together for a short time, and when cold add a pint of brandy.

❀

Drink freely of chickenweed tea or boil yarrow in milk and drink freely.

❀

A successful remedy for chronic diarrhoea: Drop eggs in water, crush a very small place in the shell to prevent bursting, then wrap in wet paper and roast in the ashes to a fine powder. It will take several hours. Sift, and take a teaspoonful of the powder three times a day.

❀

Bananas are useful as a food for those suffering from chronic diarrhoea.

For diarrhoea, parch a half pint of rice until it is perfectly brown. Boil it down as is usually done, and eat it slowly, and it will check, if not entirely stop, the most violent diarrhoea in a few hours. Ordinarily a little brandy, say half a wineglassful, with loaf sugar dissolved in it will have the same effect. However, it is better in all cases to avoid alcohol as a medicine if other antidotes can be had. In the more obstinate cases, where brandy is used, its efficacy is increased by stirring it with a red hot iron.

❀

Summer complaint is an irritation and inflammation of the lining membranes of the intestines. This may often be caused by teething, eating indigestible food, etc. If the discharges are only frequent and yellow and not accompanied with pain, there is no cause for anxiety; but if the discharges are green, soon becoming grey, brown and sometimes frothy, having a mixture of phlegm, and sometimes containing food undigested, a physician had better be summoned.

❀

In the first stages give a tablespoonful at bedtime of the following prescription: 2 oz. castor oil, 2 oz. aromatic syrup of rhubarb. This is one of the best of domestic remedies, and should always be kept on hand. Whenever the stomach of children is out of order, a dose of this simple remedy often works magic.

Dysentery

To cure dysentery mix 2 wine glasses of olive oil; 2 wineglasses molasses; 2 wine glasses rum. Simmer them well together until it becomes thick, for an hour. Stir it whilst simmering to prevent the oil separating, continue using the same till cold. Take a spoonful once an hour till the disease is abated, then once in two hours, or as the judgement may direct.

❀

Take three pints of pine bark and three pints of water, let it simmer down to a quart, strain off and add one pint West India molasses, the whole for a grown person; half for a child. This remedy is simple and effectual.

❀

Take one ounce each of laudanum, rhubarb, tincture of camphor, peppermint and red pepper. Give twenty to thirty drops every half hour until relieved. This is for adults only.

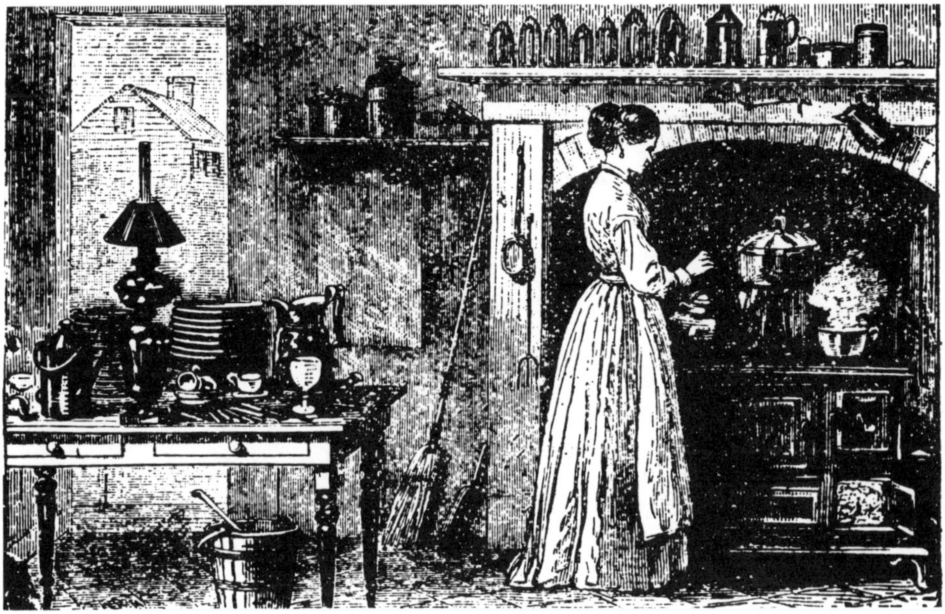

Apply woollen cloths wrung out of hot water to which a few drops of turpentine have been added. Washing out the rectum with tepid or hot water adds much to the comfort of the patient and has a curative effect. A teaspoonful of charcoal every morning and evening will produce good results.

❀

Take two quarts of ripe blackberries, a pint of loaf sugar and one-half ounce each of cinnamon, cayenne, cloves and allspice. Boil these together; strain when cold and add a pint of fourth proof brandy. According to the age, take from a tablespoonful to a wineglassful at a dose.

❀

Beat up an egg, with or without sugar, and take it as a single gulp. It seems to form a coating on the stomach and intestines, lessen inflammation and effect a speedy cure. Two or three taken during the day is generally all that is necessary. This is easily digested and is not likely to irritate.

❀

Take powdered elm bark, rhubarb and charcoal, of each half an ounce; add a tablespoonful of common salt, and the yolk of an egg, and rub the whole together well in a mortar till dry and reduced to a well-mixed powder. Give a teaspoonful three to six times a day, according to circumstances, in a little water or molasses. Valuable in dysentery or flux, and diarrhoea; seldom fails to cure.

Take good vinegar and as much salt as it will dissolve; add a tablespoonful of it to four of hot water, and let it be taken by spoonfuls as fast and hot as can be swallowed. This do once in two hours.

Indigestion and Dyspepsia

Dyspepsia may be completely cured by living for several weeks upon nothing but hard boiled eggs. The eggs should be boiled not less than 30 minutes and an hour is better. If boiled this long they are not tough but are soft and mealy. At first the patient should eat the whites only and later the yolks may also be eaten. Eat nothing else.

❀

Beat up an egg in a bowl, and then add 6 tablespoonfuls of cold water, mixing the whole well together; then add 2 tablespoonfuls of the farina (flour of) potatoes, or mashed potatoes mixing it with the liquor in the bowl: then pour in as much boiling water as will convert the whole into a jelly (like starch), and mix it well. It may be taken either alone, or with the addition of a little milk sweetened with sugar, not only for breakfast, but in cases of great debility of the stomach, or in consumptive disorders, at other meals. This dish, or food, is light, easily digested, and extremely wholesome and nourishing. Bread or biscuit should be taken with it, as the stomach gets stronger.

❀

This is a weakness in the nerves of the stomach. To cure, change your habits. If a labouring person, relax, if of sedentary habits, go to work, exercise in the open air, walk or ride.

❀

Take powdered turkey rhubarb, 2 drams; baking soda, 48 grains; simple syrup, 1 ounce; and mint water, 1/2 pint. The dose is a tablespoonful three times a day before meals. The soda is good for the gas on the stomach and the rhubarb is a laxative.

❀

Use brown bread or unbolted wheat meal, avoid condiments, saleratus, spirituous liquors—also, the violent exercise of the passion.

Drinking a cupful of hot water immediately before retiring at night and upon rising in the morning aids in the cure of dyspepsia by washing out the stomach.

In mild cases take one teaspoonful sweet oil after eating, three times a day. In severe forms take a dessertspoonful. This follow up has cured cases where doctors have given them up. Ye who suffer from this dread disease, don't fail to try it; surely it can't hurt you.

❀

There is no such thing as heartburn. What is commonly called heartburn, is nothing more nor less than acidity of the stomach, or a derangement of the digestive organs, and can be easily remedied by taking half a table-spoonful of powdered magnesia, or half a teaspoonful of saleratus, or by drinking a little lime water, or by dropping a few burning coals of hardwood in a tumbler of water, and drinking the water.

❀

Rice-water, barley-water, oatmeal-water, made by boiling a single handful of either of these to 1 qt. of water, with lemon and sugar, should be ready in every house where there are small children having dyspeptic or diarrhoeal tendencies. These drinks are surely better than cold tea, which is often given. However, milk is considered better than anything, when it is sweet and pure, and given in only small quantities at any one time, with lime-water.

❀

Many persons who think good bread and milk a luxury, frequently hesitate to eat it, for the reason that the milk will not digest readily; sourness of the stomach will often follow. But experience proves that lime-water and milk are not only food and medicine, at an early period of life, but also later when, as in the case of infants, the functions of digestion and assimilation have been seriously impaired. A stomach taxed by gluttony, irritated by improper food, inflamed by alcohol, enfeebled by disease, or otherwise unfitted for its duties—as is shown by various symptoms attendant upon indigestion, dyspepsia, diarrhoea, dysentery and fever—will resume its work, and do it energetically, on an exclusive diet of bread and milk and lime-water. A goblet of cow's milk may have 3 to 4 tablespoonfuls of lime-water added to it with good effect.

A small piece of chalk put in a pitcher of water, without imparting any taste whatever to the same, will exercise a corrective effect upon the stomachs of those who are troubled with acidity or heartburn, as it is called.

❀

Lying with the head lower than the rest of the body during sleep at night cures headache caused from a deranged stomach.

Mix some soda and ginger in the proportion of 1 teaspoonful of soda to 1/2 teaspoonful of ginger. Keep this in a tight box and take 1/2 teaspoonful in a little water before eating if digestion is bad. Soda is good for the gas and relieves the distress while the ginger is stimulating.

❀

Apples are useful in nervous dyspepsia; they are nutritious, medicinal, and vitalizing; they aid digestion, clear the voice, correct the acidity of the stomach, are valuable in rheumatism, insomnia, and liver troubles. An apple contains as much nutriment as a potato in a pleasanter and more wholesome form.

Stomach and Bowel Troubles

Ripe fruit stewed in molasses is relaxing to the bowels and a good food for the patient with stomach or bowel trouble.

❀

Warm peppermint or spearmint tea is an old tried remedy for wind on the stomach.

❀

For stomach-ache or cramps in the stomach use either essence of ginger or spirits of camphor. A mustard poultice applied to the stomach is also an excellent remedy.

❀

For inflammation of the bowels take 1 tablespoonful of spirits of turpentine and 1 tablespoonful of castor oil and beat well together, then add 1 egg and beat well together. Add 1 pint of warm water, mix it well and inject with a syringe.

❀

Wet a cloth in turpentine and lay over the part affected.

❀

Turkey corn is a good tonic for stomach or bowel troubles. Make a tea by adding 4 drams of the powdered bulb to a pint of water and give from 1 to 4 ounces 3 times a day. Or, you can use the tincture of turkey corn, from 1/2 to 1 teaspoonful doses, 3 times a day.

For inflammation of the bowels of course the safe way is to send for the doctor without delay. But in the country, one is often obliged to wait a long time. Anxiety makes the time seem long anywhere, and simple remedies are often very efficient helps. So, while you are waiting, make a paste of lard and salt, fold a wide pillow-case (as that is always at hand) into a large square, spread on the paste and lay the cloth smoothly, paste side down, over the bowels, stomach, sides and as far toward the back as you can. When the inflammation is severe, the lard will be absorbed in a very short time. Be prepared to change the paste as often as needed.

❀

A tablespoonful at bedtime, of equal parts of castor oil and aromatic syrup of rhubarb is one of the best remedies for children with stomach and bowel trouble.

Tape Worm

It is needless to attempt to give the symptoms by which the presence of worms might be distinguished; for the symptoms of nearly every other disease is, sometimes, manifested by their presence. But if the belly be quite hard and unusually large, with a peculiar and disagreeable breath in the morning, foul or furred tongue, upper lip swollen, itching of the nose and anus, milky white urine, bowels sometimes obstinately costive, then as obstinately loose, with a craving appetite, then loathing food at times; rest assured that worm medicine will not be amiss, whether the person be child, or adult. Whatever remedy may be selected, it is important that certain preparatory treatment should be adopted before the worm remedy itself is given. This treatment consists in abstinence from food for several hours, or a day; or the patient may employ light diet, such as broth and milk, for two or three days previous to the use of the remedy.

❀

Eat garlic and salt freely and every other day give a purgative of mandrake root and the worm will vacate the premises.

❀

This very annoying and distressing worm has been removed by taking two ounce doses of common pumpkin-seeds, pulverized, and repeated every four or five hours, for four or five days; spirits of turpentine, also in doses of one-half to two ounces, with castor oil have proved very effectual; the root of the male fern, valerian, bark of the pomegranate root, etc. have been used with success.

One of the commonest, and certainly a very efficient, means for expelling the worm is turpentine. This is given in quantities varying from one to two tablespoonfuls for adults, usually mixed with the same quantity of castor oil, and taken floating on milk. This dose may be repeated every second or third day, until the fragments of the worm cease to appear. The objection to the use of turpentine is that it sometimes causes difficulty in passing water, and it may induce a state of intoxication in some cases.

❀

For tape worm take sage, 1/2 pound and steep in 2 pints of water, and take a wineglassful every 3 hours. It will often be found to be effective.

❀

Blue ash bark put in a bottle of whisky and given three times a day is said to be excellent. A few drops of turpentine on loaf sugar is sometimes effective. To feed children on cooked onions several times a week, or give daily for several weeks at a time garlic bitters, will prevent them having worms.

Vomiting/Nausea/Sickness at Stomach

One of the very best remedies for nausea or vomiting is a tea made of parched corn.

❀

Much depends on the diet. If the stomach is in a restless condition, only the lightest kind of food should be taken, and it can be easily determined in a few days what food the stomach will or will not retain.

❀

Give a tablespoon of whole black mustard seed. Apply a mustard or spice plaster to the stomach.

❀

A tea made of peppermint, spearmint or ginger will generally relieve vomiting. Brandy or tincture of ginger are other remedies that are much used.

❀

Take an ounce each of powdered ginger, cinnamon, cloves and black pepper and a dram of pulverized cayenne; mix, and add a fluid ounce of tincture of ginger and enough honey to make a thick paste. When applied over the stomach this is excellent for sickness at the stomach and vomiting.

Steep some chickweed and drink of it to stop vomiting.

❀

Make a strong tea of cloves or of ginger and cloves and give the patient a little every 5 or 10 minutes.

❀

If the bowels are hot and feverish, bind a cold compress upon the belly over night, covering it well with flannel. The warm bath should be used twice a week. The diet must be of the most simple, unirritating kind—beginning with a solution of gum arabic, rice-water, barley-water, arrowroot or sago gruel, and gradually rising as the symptoms improve, to beef tea, mutton and chicken broth, tender beef steak, etc.

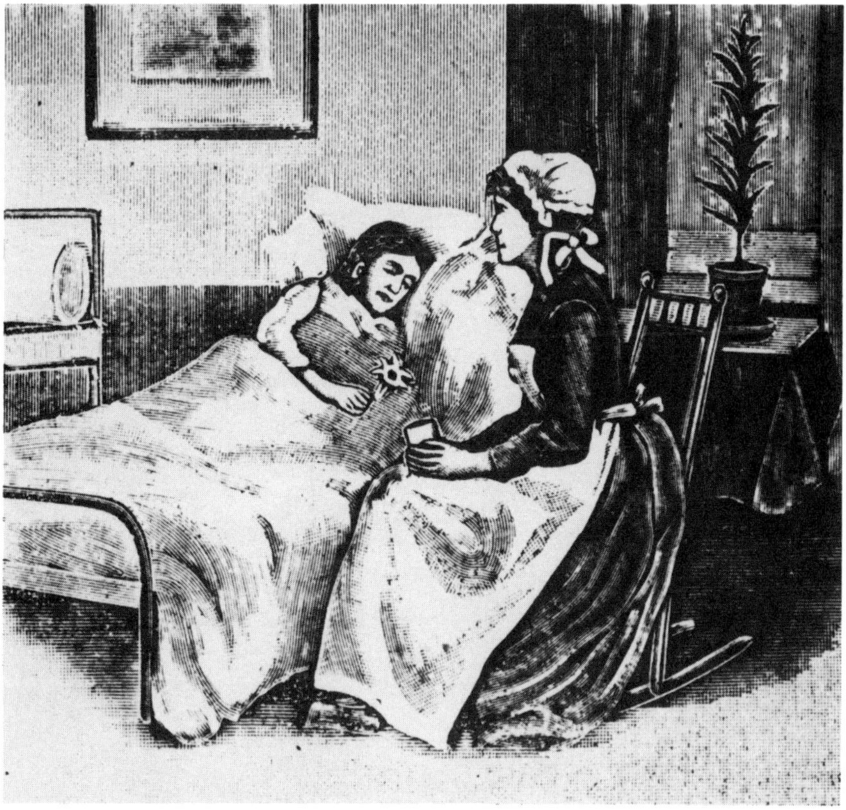

Nervous Disorders

Headaches

For a sick headache drink a cup of coffee to which has been added the juice of a lemon or 2 tablespoonfuls of vinegar.

❀

The *Medical Record* is authority for the statement that nervous headache may be cured by the simple act of walking backwards for ten minutes. It is well to get in a long, narrow room where the windows are high, and walk very slowly, placing first the ball of the foot on the floor, and then the heel. Besides curing the headache, this exercise promotes a graceful carriage.

❀

Put one ounce of bromide of potash in four ounces of water. Take one teaspoon in half a cup of water.

❀

Coarse brown paper soaked in vinegar and placed on the forehead is good for a sick headache. If the eyelids are gently bathed in cool water the pain in the head is generally allayed.

❀

Persons subject to headache will find a perfect relief by taking a cold shower bath every morning.

❀

A remedy for headache due to digestive disorders is the exercise of regularity and moderation in eating, with an avoidance of food which is innutritious and difficult of digestion, and attention to the regularity of the bowels. The last point is of special importance.

❀

A mixture of ice and salt, in proportion of one to one-half, applied to the head, frequently gives instant relief from acute headache. It should be tied up in a small linen cloth, like a pad, and held as near as possible to the seat of the pain.

❀

Mix a tablespoonful of cayenne pepper to a thick paste with vinegar, spread it on a strip of thin cloth, which may be folded together, and bind on the forehead from temple to temple. Then swallow a "pinch" of the pepper—say a quarter of a teaspoonful—in a teaspoonful of vinegar or lemon juice. The plaster will burn but not blister, and in the course of ten minutes the headache will disappear under the stimulating effect of this treatment.

❀

Nervous headache is said to be instantly relieved by shampooing the head with a quart of cold water in which a dessertspoonful of soda has been dissolved.

❀

Add a teaspoonful of lemon juice to 2 gills of warm water. Repeat this dose every 15 minutes. Hundreds of cases of sick headache are cured with this simple remedy. Let it become more generally known and there will be much less suffering from this sickness.

❀

Look for cause, and remove it if possible. Regulate the diet and keep the bowels in good condition. Plenty of out-door exercise with freedom from care, will prevent the attacks. For a throbbing headache, with flushed face, apply cold water or ice bag to the head. Hot foot bath and inhalation of camphor, or mustard plaster on back of neck. For headache with pallor of face, and faintness on standing, apply hot water to the head freely, and inhalation of ammonia will often relieve.

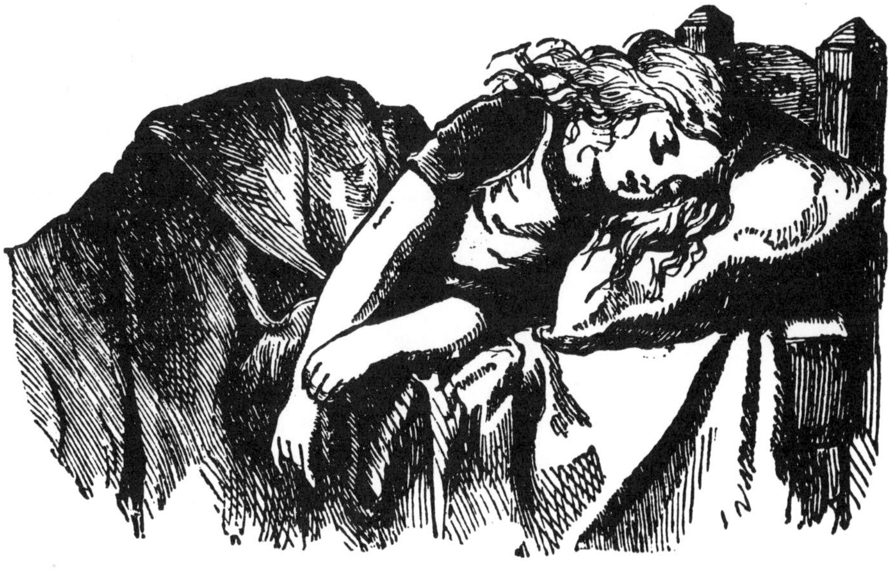

To cure sick headache arising from acidity, all that is necessary is to soak the feet in hot water about twenty minutes, drinking at the same time some of the herb-teas, such as pennyroyal, catnip, or mint, etc., then get into bed, cover up warm and keep up a sweating process for about an hour, by which time relief will have been obtained.

❀

If the headache is caused by congestion of blood in the head, bathe the head with vinegar and cold water and the feet with warm water. Bathe the temples and forehead with either warm or cold water as desired.

❀

For a sick headache, two teaspoonfuls of finely powdered charcoal, drunk in half a tumbler of water, will often give relief to the headache, when caused, as in most cases it is, by a superabundance of acid in the stomach.

Neuralgia (painful affliction of the nerves) and Nervous Troubles

Nervous people should eat fat food. Every irritable and exhaustive nerve should, if possible, be coated with fat. Fat is to a tender nerve what an air cushion is to a tired invalid—it eases jolts wonderfully. With the fat should be combined grain foods and vegetables for strength, and fruits to keep up a healthful consistency of the blood.

❀

A hot bath, a stroll in the fresh air, shampooing the head in weak soda-water, or a timely nap in a cool, quiet room will sometimes stop a nervous headache. When overfatigued from shopping or sightseeing a sponge dipped in very hot water and pressed repeatedly over the back of the neck between the ears will be found exceedingly refreshing, especially if the face and temples are afterward subjected to the same treatment. Neuralgia is caused not only by cold air, but by acidity of the stomach, starved nerves, imperfect teeth, or by indolence combined with a too generous diet.

❀

A noted cure for neuralgia is hot vinegar vapourized. Heat a flat-iron sufficiently hot to vapourize the vinegar, cover this with some woollen material, which is moistened with vinegar, and the apparatus is then applied at once to the painful spot. The application may be repeated until the pain disappears.

Many cases of neuralgia have been cured by the common field thistle. The leaves are macerated and used on the parts affected as a poultice, while a small quantity of the leaves are made a tea of, and a small wine of the decoction is taken as a drink before each meal.

❀

Thicken the yolk of an egg with salt, and apply as a poultice. Raw onions sliced and mixed with shavings of common hard soap and applied often gives relief to neuralgia and toothache.

❀

Horseradish is an excellent remedy for neuralgia. Grate the horseradish and mix it with vinegar the same as when it is intended for the table. Apply this to the temple when the neuralgia is in the face and to the wrist when it is in the arm or shoulder.

❀

Mix salt and ashes, heat well, put into a salt bag and apply to the parts affected with neuralgia.

❀

An external application of peppermint is highly recommended. Eat plenty of fat meat, and avoid tea, but drink plenty of milk. Avoid exposure to dampness.

❀

Bathe the feet for half an hour in hot mustard water and at the same time drink smartweed tea; or, ginger tea will do. Then go to bed and take a sweat for from half to three-quarters of an hour. After the sweat, sponge the body with warm water, dry, and rub briskly with the hands. This is good for neuralgia which comes from a cold or from inflammation.

❀

Heat is the best and quickest cure for this distressing pain. A hot flat-iron, passed rapidly and deftly over several folds of flannel laid on the affected spot, will often give relief in less than ten minutes, without the aid of medicine. Hot fomentations are of equal value; though when the skin is very tender it is more advisable to use dry heat, nothing being better for the purpose than bags of heated salt, flour or sand, which retain warmth for a long time.

❀

Hot fomentations of hops generally give relief from neuralgia.

Skin

Baldness and Dandruff

Onions must be rubbed frequently on the part. The stimulating powers of this vegetable are of essential service in restoring the tone of the skin, and assisting the capillary vessels in sending forth new hair; but it is not infallible. Should it succeed, however, the growth of these new hairs may be assisted by the oil of myrtleberries, the repute of which, perhaps, is greater than its real efficiency. These applications are cheap and harmless, even where they do no good; a character which cannot be said of the numerous quack remedies that meet the eye in every direction.

❀

Put equal quantities of rum and sweet oil into a bottle, and, before using, shake them well together. This mixture should be applied with a soft brush to the roots of the hair every night; it should be tried for a month at the least, before any improvement can be expected.

❀

Three grains of tartaric acid, a few drops of lemon juice, in six ounces of soft water, with this wet the head two or three times a week. The skin will be soft and the hair firm.

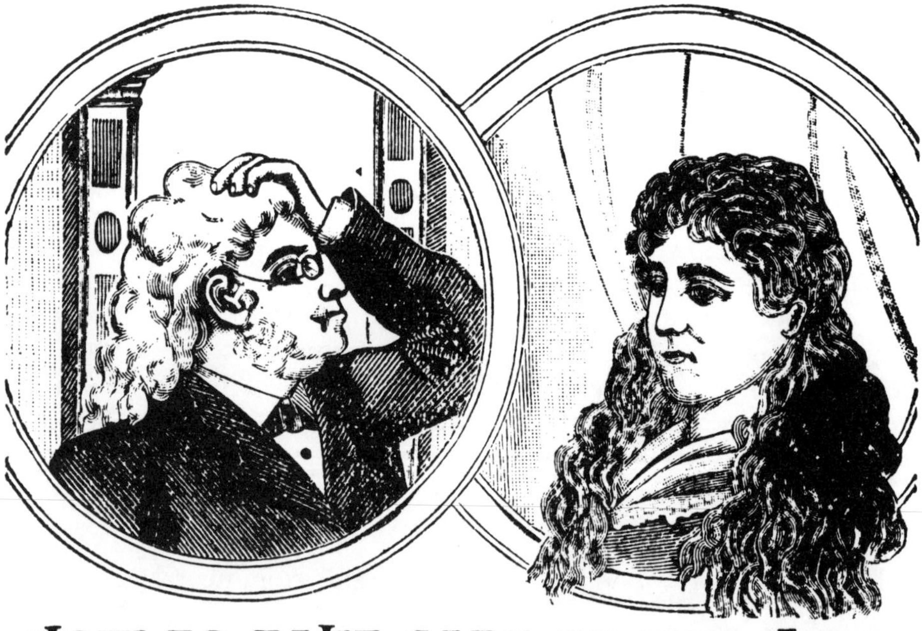

HOW TO TAKE CARE OF THE HAIR.

To prevent hair from falling out or turning grey, take a teacupful of dried sage, and boil it in a quart of soft water for twenty minutes. Strain it off and add a piece of borax the size of a walnut; pulverize the borax. Put the sage tea, when cool, into a quart bottle; add the borax; shake well together, and keep in a cool place. Brush the hair thoroughly and rub the wash well on the head with the hand. Then, after a good hard rubbing, brush the hair well before the fire so it will become dry.

❀

To increase the growth of hair, take of mutton suet, one pound; best white wax, four ounces; essences of bergamot and lemon, of each, three drams; oils of lavender and thyme, of each, one dram. Mix the suet and wax over a gentle fire and then add the perfumes.

❀

A shampoo with raw egg will remove all the dandruff.

❀

For dandruff wash the head with a mixture composed of an ounce each of borax and camphor and a pint and a half of cold water. After each washing run in a little pure olive oil.

❀

As a good hair oil, take 1 pint olive oil and heat it to 200 degrees in a pan (not iron); add 1/2 oz. of pearl ash. Stir well for 10 minutes, let it cool and then filter.

❀

To thicken hair take one quart of white wine, one handful of rosemary flowers, one half pound of honey, one quarter pint of oil of sweet almonds. Mix the rosemary and honey with the wine, distill them together, then add the oil of sweet almonds and shake well. When using it, pour a little into a cup, warm it, and rub it into the roots of the hair.

❀

Take of lard one tablespoonful and rub in a quarter of a teaspoonful of tar (not coal tar, but pine tar). Rub this salve well into the scalp every night, and by morning the disagreeable odour will be gone.

❀

To prevent the hair from falling out apply once a week a wash made of one quart of boiling water, one ounce of pulverized borax and half an ounce of powdered camphor. Rub on with a sponge or a piece of flannel.

To a pint of water add 1 gill of onion juice and one ounce of pearl ash and wash the hair with the solution.

❀

Make some sage tea and rub on the scalp every night for one week; then wash the hair and repeat. It is claimed this will grow hair as well as prevent its falling.

❀

Rub a little olive oil into the scalp every 4 or 5 days.

❀

For a hair restorative take of black mustard seed 1/2 oz., red pepper 15 grains, blood root 1/2 oz., cantharides 15 grains, castile soap 1/2 oz., alcohol one quart; mix all together in a bottle, let stand for a week, occasionally shaking. Perfume with oil of bergamot, and apply three or four times a day.

❀

The best method of promoting the growth of whiskers and moustaches, is to shave the parts frequently, and use as a stimulant the ashes of burned tobacco macerated in bay water.

❀

To restore hair use alcohol, 1 pint; rain water, 1 pint; aqua ammonia, 1 ounce. Mix, wet the head thoroughly and rub well to the roots of the hair daily, will be found the best in the world. This was sold many times for $5.00.

❀

If your hair is falling out, rub slices of lemon thoroughly into the roots and over the scalp. Will cure dandruff, and preserves and strengthens the roots of the hair.

Boils

After opening the boil thoroughly, and squeezing out all the pus, apply a warm poultice for a day, and then wash with castile soap or boracic acid, and dress it with soft linen until well.

❀

A poultice of camomile flowers will draw a boil to a head so that it may be opened. It holds heat and moisture for a long time and it has a sedative, or quieting and soothing, action on the local parts which is due to its oily constituents.

Apply a flaxseed or linseed meal poultice. This retains heat and moisture for a long time.

❀

Take 1 cupful of corn meal, 2 large onions cut up fine, and 2 ounces of laundry soap; mix, and apply as a hot poultice. This poultice not only has heat and moisture, which are desired, but the soap and onions have drawing power.

❀

These should be brought to a head by warm poultices of boiled white lily root, or onion root by fermentation with hot water, or by stimulating plasters. When ripe they should be destroyed by a needle or lancet; but this should not be attempted until they are fully proved.

Bunions/Corns

To cure this pestiferous and painful sore, soak the part in warm water for one hour, with a razor shave off all the dead parts to the quick, take a bit of brown diaculum, as large as a pea, place it on the corn with a bit of cloth over it. They will both stick without further attention. Wear a loose shoe and the corn will certainly get well.

❀

When the bunion is painful, put three or four leeches on the joint of the toe, and do not disturb them till they drop off; then bathe the bunions twice a day in fresh cream, and afterward renounce tight boots. Of course this remedy will not remove the swelling of the bone.

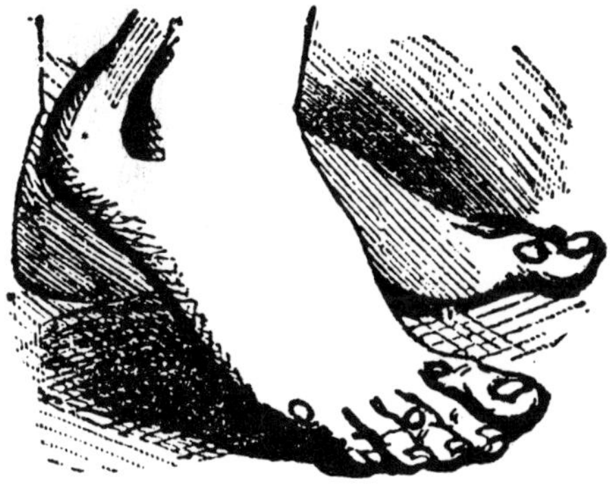

HOW TO CURE CORNS, CHILBLAINS, INGROWING NAILS, COLD FEET, ETC.

If a cripple will take a lemon, cut off a piece, then nick it so as to let in the toe with the corn, the pulp next to the corn—tie this on at night, so that it cannot move—he will find next morning that, with a blunt knife, the corn will come away to a great extent.

❀

Boil some tobacco to make an extract, mix with white pine pitch and apply to the corn. Renew once a week until the corn is gone.

❀

Soak some bran in cider vinegar and bind on the corn for three nights.

❀

Mix vaseline with camphor and apply frequently.

❀

Let fall a stream of very warm water from a tea-kettle, at the highest elevation from which the patient can bear the water to fall directly on the apex of the swelling: continue this once a day for a short time and a cure will be effected, providing you desist from wearing short shoes. The greater the elevation of the kettle, the more effectual the remedy.

❀

Wrapping a piece of linen wet in turpentine about the toe night and morning will cure soft corns.

❀

Boil a potato in its skin, and after it is boiled take the skin and put the inside of it to the corn, and leave it on for about twelve hours; at the end of that period the corn will be nearly cured.

❀

To cure corns soak some bread in vinegar for 2 days and put a piece as a cold poultice on the corn overnight, binding it on with a strip of rag. Every 3 days soak the feet in hot water and peel off a layer of the corn. Continue the treatment until the corn has entirely disappeared.

❀

Take half a teacup of vinegar and thicken with light breadcrumbs. Apply as a poultice. Sliced lemon bound to the corn is effective.

❀

Pine pitch, or pine tar, as some call it, brown sugar and saltpetre, each, 1 teaspoonful. Simmer together. Pare the corn as close as you can. Spread some of the salve on an old kid glove or other thin, soft leather, the size of the corn; bind it on for 2 or 3 days; when taken off the corn comes off with it.

❀

Take equal parts brown sugar, yellow soap, mix to a salve then soften with coal-oil. Put vaseline around corn to prevent blistering . Apply salve to corn and tie on with a rag. When salve becomes hard, put on fresh salve. Do this until corn is ready to be removed.

Burns/Scalds

Smear the scorched surface with glycerine, by means of a feather, then apply cotton wadding; lastly, cover with oil-silk.

❀

Equal parts of cod liver oil and chloroform used as a liniment will relieve the pain of burns.

❀

For burns and scalds nothing is more soothing than the white of an egg, which may be poured over the wound. It is softer as a varnish for a burn than collodion, and being always at hand can be applied immediately. It is also more cooling than the sweet oil and cotton which was formerly supposed to be the surest application to allay the smarting pain. It is the contact with the air which gives the extreme discomfort experienced from the ordinary accident of this kind, and anything which excludes the air and prevents inflammation is the thing to be applied.

❀

Put 1 pint linseed oil, 1/2 pint lime water and the yolks of 2 eggs in a bottle and shake well. Soak cotton wool with the preparation and apply. Bind on with a bandage.

❀

Take some freshly gathered lavender buds and crush them well. Mix 1 lb. of pulp with 1 1/2 lb. of unsalted lard. Boil slowly for a few minutes, stirring well. Pour into small pots and tie down. If applied at once when the burn occurs, no pain will be felt.

❀

Take fresh lard, any quantity, and work into it a quantity of powdered soot—about a tablespoonful of soot to an ounce of lard—and apply. This is one of the best applications for burns and scalds that can be made.

Equal parts of turpentine, sweet oil, and beeswax; melt the oil and wax together, and when a little cool, add the turpentine, and stir until cold, which keeps them evenly mixed. Apply by spreading upon thin cloth—linen is the best. This is a good salve for burns, frost-bites, cracked nipples, etc.

❀

Take a tart apple, and simmer in lard until it forms a salve. It will then heal a burn quickly and always without a scar.

❀

It has been found that wheat flour is an excellent remedy for burns. It is to be sprinkled on so as to completely cover the wound or burnt part; it protects the part from the atmosphere, exposure to which is one great cause of the pain. It also draws out the fire. The wound may also be bathed at the same time, just previous to applying the flour, with limewater and sweet oil, equal parts, by means of a feather.

❀

A superficial burn covering a large surface is often more dangerous than a deep one, confined to a small place. If there is any cause for apprehension of danger, send for a physician at once. If prostration or fainting is produced by the shock a little brandy should be given until there is a revival of strength. Should a burn be slight, cold water applied freely will give relief. When the pain has moderated a dressing of hog's lard is good, or the white of an egg beaten, and spread thick over the burn. Soap from the shaving cup applied with a brush sometimes gives relief. A simple and effective remedy for a burn, is a saturated solution of bi-carbonate of soda, in either plain or camphorated water. Keep the burn covered with soft rags thoroughly wet until the pain subsides.

❀

For burns, sweet oil and cotton are the standard remedies. If they are not at hand sprinkle the burned part with flour and wrap loosely with a soft cloth. Don't remove the dressing until the inflammation subsides, as it will break the new skin that is forming.

❀

Soak a piece of linen rag in linseed oil, suspend it from the tongs over a saucer, and ignite the lower end; the oil which drops from it, while consuming, should be applied, when cold, with a feather, to the burn or scald.

❀

A burn or scald is always painful; but the pain can be instantly relieved by the use of bi-carbonate of soda, or common baking soda (saleratus).

Put two tablespoonfuls of soda in a half cup of water. Wet a piece of linen cloth in the solution and lay it on the burn. The pain will disappear as if by magic. If the burn is so deep that the skin has peeled off, dredge the dry soda directly on the part affected.

❀

Saturate a soft piece of fabric with alcohol, lay it over the burn, then cover it with cotton or finely picked oakum. This is the most clean dressing that can be adapted. It may be thought that alcohol applied to a burn will produce more pain; but try it, and you will be agreeably surprised to observe how quickly it will allay the pain. Subsequently disturb the dressing as little as possible; wet the dressing occasionally with alcohol, and the result you will find better than by any other method.

Freckles

Mix two ounces of rectified spirits of wine, add two teaspoonfuls of muriatic acid, with one pound and a half of distilled water.

❀

Wash the face every morning in fresh buttermilk, then rinse in warm water and dry with a soft towel.

❀

One of the best things for freckles is to apply sour buttermilk at night, let it dry on the face and wash off in the morning.

❀

In order to remove freckles, apply at night a mixture of equal parts of strained lemon juice, glycerine, olive oil and curdled milk.

❀

Crush some strawberries and rub them over the face at night just before going to bed.

❀

Take the juice of a cucumber pressed from the fruit. Boil over a quick fire, cool rapidly and bottle. Apply a tablespoonful diluted with two tablespoonfuls of water, night and morning. Or, juice of horse-radish 1/2 pint; cider vinegar 1 pint. Mix and apply night and morning.

❀

Bruise and squeeze the juice out of common chickweed, and to this juice add three times its quantity of soft water. Bathe the skin with this for five or ten minutes morning and evening, and wash afterwards with clean water. Elder flowers treated and applied exactly in the same manner as above. When the flowers are not to be had, the distilled water from them, which may be procured from any druggist, will answer the purpose.

❀

Take beef's gall one ounce; saleratus, borax and gum guaiac, of each half an ounce, pulverized; alcohol and rose or rain-water, of each half a pint; mix, and let stand ten days, shaking occasionally. Use as a wash twice a day.

❀

Put into a bottle 1/2 dram of powdered borax, 1 dram of sugar and 2 ounces of lemon juice. Let stand for several days, then rub the face three times daily.

❀

At night use the following ointment: 1 oz. white wax; 1 teacupful of nice white lard; lump of camphor, the size of a chestnut; 1 teaspoonful of glycerine. Put the wax and camphor in a tin to melt, crumbling the camphor; when melted, add the other ingredients. Stir thoroughly, and pour into molds which have been dipped in water.

❀

Let some grated horseradish stand for five hours in some very sour milk. Use this as a wash every night and morning.

❀

Freckles are always developed on the parts of body most exposed to the sun, and on some persons disappear in winter. They seldom appear on children before the age of five, and usually disappear in old age. Mix 4 ounces of rose water; 40 grains of borax; 1/4 ounce of dilute acetic acid; 6 grains of corrosive sublimate. Apply with a soft brush or rag every morning and evening, and continue until the freckles disappear. Avoid the sun as much as possible during the treatment. Avoid all blistering compounds.

❀

Mix bitter almonds and barley flour in equal parts. Apply in the form of a paste.

The Itch

This arises from insects (animalculae) which insinuate themselves beneath the skin, and produce festers. Sulphur is a poison to these insects. Take hog's lard, four parts and melt it; add to the melted lard one part of sulphur. Apply this ointment five or six nights and it will cure, drink yellow dock root tea for the blood. Yellow dock ointment is acure also.

❀

Take 2 drams sulphur; 2 drams bay-berries, in powder; 2 drams sulphate of zinc; 20 drops essence of Bergamot; and olive oil sufficient to make the mass into an ointment. To be rubbed on the parts affected every night and washed off in the morning—this ointment is said to be very effective and safe.

❀

Take sulphate of potash one ounce, water one pint, sulphuric acid half an ounce; mix. Bathe the parts affected with the disease twice a day with this lotion, first washing the parts well with soap and water. Change the clothes often and keep the parts as clean as possible.

❀

Keep the bowels open and regular. Take flower of sulphur and lard or fresh butter enough to make a good ointment and anoint the body all over every night before retiring. Wash thoroughly with warm water every morning. For an itch ointment take 1 pound unsalted butter; 2 ounces

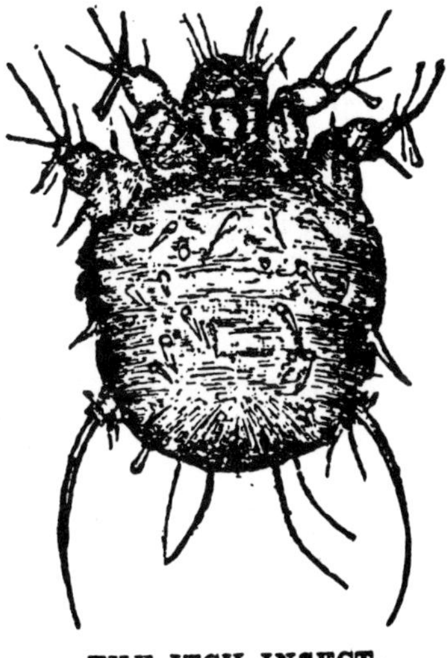

THE ITCH INSECT.

How to Cure the Itch.

burgundy pitch; 1 dram powdered saltpetre; 1 pint powdered sulphur. Melt, and mix thoroughly together and apply every evening.

❀

Take fine sulphur, one ounce, turpentine, one ounce, lard half a pound, melt the lard and turpentine, then add the sulphur, stir it till cold—apply it two or three times a day. It soon cures the complaint without changing the clothes.

❀

For the itch, wash the parts affected with strong rum.

Sunburn and Tan

This is fine for burns, scalds and sunburns. Mix and shake well equal parts of lime water, camphor and linseed oil.

❀

To remove tan mix lemon juice, 1/2 ounce; new milk, 1/2 pint; brandy, 1/2 ounce. Boil and skim off the scum. Apply every night and morning. Or, take a lemon, cut it in two, and rub it over the face. Wash it off and apply magnesia moistened in water and let it dry on the face. When dry, wash it off. Repeat this three or four times successively.

❀

Put a few drops of cologne into some elder flower tea and bathe the face for sunburn.

❀

Cold fresh cream frequently applied will remove sunburn.

❀

Slice some cucumbers and let them stand in water for some time. Wash the face and hands with this water.

❀

.The following wash is much employed for removing sunburn and whitening the skin. Mix fresh horseradish root, 1 oz; cold buttermilk, 1 pint. Put aside for four hours, then use as a wash. Or take of, the juice of horseradish, 1 part; cider vinegar, 2 parts. Mix. This is also recommended for removing freckles.

❀

Apply lemon juice for sunburn.

Wash the face before retiring with buttermilk and in the morning wash with weak bran tea with a little cologne added.

Warts

To destroy warts apply a mixture of chromic acid and water, equal parts, or an application of carbolic or nitric acid will have the same effect, or rub the warts night and morning with sal ammoniac moistened in water. This will remove them in a short time.

❀

Mix thoroughly half an ounce of sulphur with the same quantity of alcohol and apply freely once or twice a day.

❀

Burn some common willow bark, mix the ashes with strong vinegar and apply frequently to the affected part.

❀

To cure warts, take half an ounce of sulphur, half an ounce of 90% spirits, put into an ounce phial, shake them well together, then freely apply to the affected parts, for a few days, once or twice a day, and in a few weeks or months at most the warts will disappear.

❀

A phial of water made very sour with tartaric acid, applied to the warts often for a few days, and they will certainly go off.

❀

Bruise milkweeds and apply the milk that runs from them to the warts several times a day and they will soon come off.

❀

Boil some potatoes, and with the water in which they are boiled, bathe the warts. At the end of a week they will have nearly, if not quite, gone.

❀

Cut a piece of wild turnip, from the woods, and rub several times upon the wart or warts.

❀

Warts can be removed by steeping or soaking a small piece of beef all night in vinegar. Cut what will cover the wart and tie it on with strips of sticking plaster. Take meat off in a days time and put back on at night. In two weeks, the warts will die and fall off.

Colds and the Lungs

Asthma

Take a tea made by steeping white poplar bark in water. The dose is half a wineglassful.

❀

Relief is often obtained by applying a strong mustard poultice over the stomach and chest. Mustard irritates, causing the tubes to dilate and thus aids the breathing.

❀

The following mixture is recommended as a relief for the asthmatic. Two ounces of the best honey, and one ounce of castor oil mixed. A teaspoonful to be taken night and morning.

❀

An excellent remedy is to take a teaspoonful of powdered alum mixed with a little molasses every 15 minutes until it causes vomiting.

❀

As a common drink, a tea made of the leaves of common chestnut, which had fallen from the tree in autumn; sweeten well, and continue its use for 2 or 3 months.

❀

Take a cupful of vinegar; add a wineglassful of turpentine and 1 egg; beat together and use as a liniment on the chest.

❀

A general treatment for asthma is to protect the chest with warm clothing. Do not sleep on, or handle, beds or pillows made either of feathers or straw but use a corn husk mattress and husk or air pillow. Do not use straw matting in the house or straw under the carpets. There seems to be small particles flying from matting and straw that irritate the air passages. Use every precaution against taking cold. Discard corsets and do not wear low necked dresses. Never sit down or lie down with damp feet. Keep the feet warm and the nerves quiet.

❀

Those suffering from asthma should eat only easily digested food. Eat light suppers and avoid catching cold. Shower baths every morning are highly recommended if the patient is sufficiently strong. Drinking strong

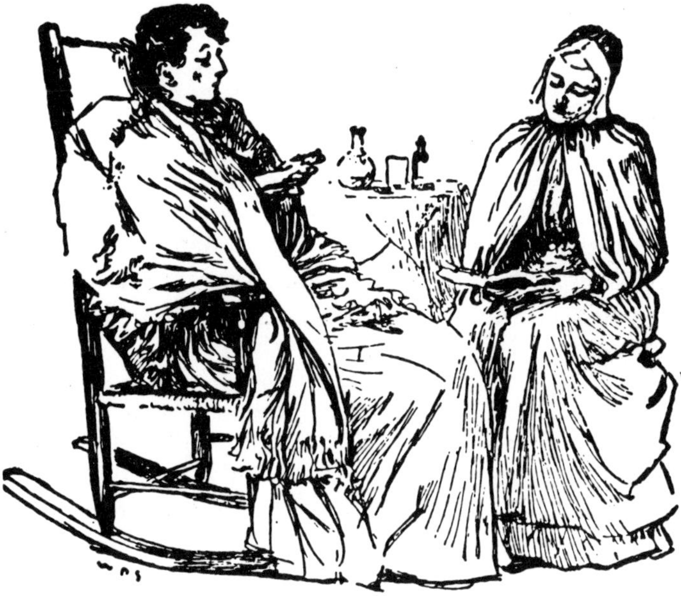

READING TO THE SICK.

coffee is sometimes a great relief in a fit of asthma. Burning nitre-paper and inhaling the fumes is very effective. Smoking jimson-weed (thorn-apple) is an excellent remedy in some cases. Keep the bowels open.

❀

Cut up four or five bulbs of Indian turnip, put in a quart of whisky. Dose, a tablespoon three times a day. The bottle can be refilled several times. This is an excellent remedy, which those who have asthma should test. Be careful in procuring the root, as there is a poisonous plant of similar appearance.

❀

For asthma take 1 oz. of camomile flowers; 2 oz. of Irish moss; 1 oz of Virginia snake root; 2 oz. of licorice root. Boil together in 1 gallon of water till reduced to half a gallon. Give 1 tablepoonful 3 times a day before meals.

❀

Gather some leaves from the mullein plant and soak them overnight in saltpetre water, then dry and crumble to a powder. Place in a saucer and light. The smoke from this must be inhaled and makes breathing much easier.

Bronchitis

For either simple or chronic bronchitis take a teaspoonful of petroleum before each meal.

❀

For the cough of bronchitis give an adult a teaspoonful of thc following mixture 3 or 4 times a day. Mix 1 ounce each of lemon juice, sweet spirits of nitre, olive oil and honey. Lemon juice and honey are good for the cough. The nitre works on the kidneys and the castor oil on the bowels and casts off waste material.

❀

Let the patient breathe the steam from hot catnip or horehound tea. Steam is soothing to the inflamed surfaces and so also are the fumes of catnip and horehound. The horehound is also an expectorant.

❀

Take a small piece of saltpetre—as large as half a pea and put in your mouth and let it dissolve once a day.

❀

Give a teaspoonful of the tincture of skunk cabbage 4 times a day for bronchitis and asthma.

❀

Get from the druggist's a little good wood creosote. Put two drops of it into a bottle holding a pint or so. Pour in a little more than half a pint of clear water, and shake it well; shake well always before using it. Take a mouthful of this, throw the head back, gargle it some time in the throat, and then swallow it. Repeat this every two hours, more or less, so as to use up the liquid within twenty-four hours. For each subsequent twenty-four hours, use three drops of the creosote in three to four gills of water. This three drops a day may be continued as long as any bronchitis appears. Two to four days is usually enough, though it may be continued indefinitely without harm.

Colds, Coughs and Hoarseness

To cure a cold before retiring, soak the feet in mustard water as hot as can be endured, the feet should at first be plunged in a pail half full of lukewarm water, adding by degrees very hot water until the desired heat is attained, protecting the body and knees with blankets so as to direct the vapour from the water to induce a good sweat. Next, to 2 tablespoonfuls of boiling water, add 1 tablespoonful of white sugar and 14 drops of strong spirits of camphor. Drink the whole and cuddle in bed under plenty of bedclothes and sleep it off.

❀

For a cough syrup, boil four lemons until soft, slice, and put in a quart cup with a pound of cream candy; stir twenty minutes, when cool, add one tablespoon of sweet almonds. Dose, one tablespoon whenever the cough is troublesome.

❀

For coughs, an excellent home preparation is made as follows: Boil a tablespoonful of liquid tar in a quart of rain water; strain through a cheese-cloth; place again over the fire; add a pound of horehound candy, a cup of granulated sugar and a half a spoonful of pulverized alum.

❀

Boil one ounce each of anise-seed and licorice stick, with half an ounce of senna, in one quart of water; strain and add two cups of honey, boil down to a pint and bottle.

❀

For cold in the lungs make a poultice of onions fried in lard and lay on the chest. Soak the feet in as hot water as can be borne and drink a glass of hot lemonade and, if you have it, a little senna tea before going to bed. Lemonade will cause sweating, senna will move the bowels and the onions will loosen the cold by drawing the congestion from the lungs.

❀

Horseradish steeped in vinegar, sweetened with honey, is excellent; when a cough is severe, a teaspoonful every twenty minutes.

❀

To cure a cold without medicine, wrap up very warm in bed, with a hot iron to the feet; drink any warm tea, or take a vinegar stew to produce a mild perspiration. In the morning take a warm sponge bath. Keep the bowels open, and use a light diet.

❀

Wet ground mustard with the white of an egg—spread it on a cloth—and apply till the skin reddens. Extraordinary to ease pain, and inflammation.

❀

Take 1/2 pint of whisky, 4 ounces of glycerine and 1 ounce of rock candy. The dose is a teaspoonful three or four times a day or when the cough is troublesome.

Eat a hot roasted onion or onion syrup before going to bed. The onion is a fine thing for colds.

❀

Doses of oil, cod-liver oil, skunk's oil, goose grease, and many other sorts, have been found to help certain persons when suffering from colds but not all. It is probably a question of digesting them or not. But whatever further medication one may elect, do not let it divert attention from the one greatest remedy—cold, pure air.

❀

When the cold seems to have made the lungs its special point of attack, apply a mustard plaster mixed with the white of an egg, to draw the irritation to the surface as quickly as possible; then follow with a poultice of cooked linseed oil meal. If this does not afford relief, call the doctor, for the case is a serious one.

❀

Put five cents' worth of pine pitch into a pint of water. Let it simmer until the water is well impregnated with the flavour. Dip out the gum which remains undissolved and add honey enough to sweeten and make a thick syrup. Strain this and bottle. Take a teaspoonful four or five times a day, according to the severity of the cough. It will afford speedy relief.

❀

Take garlic juice. The dose is half a dram. This is also good for nervous and spasmodic coughs in children. The bruised bulbs, applied as a poultice on the chest and spine, are very good for children with pneumonia.

❀

Heat together some honey and vinegar and melt a little fresh butter in the mixture. Take one or two teaspoonfuls as often as necessary for a cough.

❀

Hard raisins cut in pieces and fine-cut tobacco, equal parts; simmer together, strain and press out all the dregs. This is excellent for cold in the head, applied to the nose and temples; also for croup, rubbed on the throat and chest.

❀

Sometimes a sore throat can be cured by the following simple recipe: Soak in water a small piece of bread and mix with it a pinch of cayenne pepper; roll it up in the form of a pill and swallow it. Usually in three hours the patient will be relieved of all pain. In aggravated cases a second dose may be requisite.

❀

Almost instant relief may be had in the case of cold in the head, by a rigid and systematic practice of open air exercise and inhaling long breaths of fresh air four or five times a day. This practice, in conjunction with a spare diet and occasionally skipping a meal altogether, will cure almost any cold in the head if taken in the first stage of the disease.

❀

Take 1/4 ounce each of camphor, spirits of turpentine, aqua ammonia and sweet oil and apply externally for cold in the chest, neuralgia, sore throat and rheumatism. For external use only.

❀

To a pint and a half of water, add two large poppy-heads, and two large lemons. Boil them till they are soft, press the lemons into the water, strain the liquor, and add half a dram of saffron, and half a pound of brown sugar-candy, pounded. Boil all together till the sugar-candy is dissolved; stir the whole till you perceive it will jelly; strain it a second time, and take the seeds from the poppies.

❀

Borax has proved a most effective remedy in certain forms of colds. In sudden hoarseness or loss of voice in public speakers or singers, from colds, relief for an hour or so may be obtained by slowly dissolving, and partially swallowing, a lump of borax the size of a garden pea, or about three or four grains held in the mouth for ten or fifteen minutes before speaking or singing. This produces a profuse secretion of saliva, or "watering" of the mouth and throat, just as wetting brings back the missing notes to a flute when it is too dry.

❀

A flannel dipped in boiling water and sprinkled with turpentine, laid on the chest as quickly as possible, will relieve the most severe cold or hoarseness.

❀

A remedy for winter coughs is to mix equal parts lemon juice, honey and cod liver oil together, and take a tablespoonful of the mixture whenever the cough is troublesome. It is better to make a small quantity at a time. For children give a teaspoonful.

Take four ounces of grated fresh horseradish, saturate it in a pint of good vinegar over night, then add half a pint of honey, and bring it to the boiling point; then strain and squeeze out. Take one or two teaspoonfuls several times a day. Very good for hoarseness, loss of voice, and all ordinary coughs.

❀

Keep the bowels open with castor oil and molasses and grease the nostrils with mutton suet, sweet oil or lard.

❀

Take a large teacupful of linseed, two pennyworth of stick liquorice, and quarter of a pound of sun raisins. Put these into two quarts of soft water, and let it simmer over a slow fire till it is reduced to one; then add to it a quarter of a pound of brown sugar-candy (pounded), a tablespoonful of old rum, and a tablespoonful of the best white-wine vinegar, or lemon-juice. Drink half a pint at going to bed, and take a little when the cough is troublesome. This receipt generally cures the worst of colds in two or three days, and if taken in time, may be said to be almost an infallible remedy.

❀

Inflammation of the throat can be cured by applying powdered alum to the affected part with the finger. This never fails to cure if applied before an abscess is formed in the tonsils.

❀

To cure a cold take: 1 tablespoonful of molasses; 2 teaspoonfuls castor oil; 1 teaspoonful paregoric; 1 teaspoonful spirits of camphor. Mix them and take it often.

❀

For hoarseness take the white of 2 eggs and beat them with 2 spoonfuls of white sugar. Grate in a little nutmeg, then add a pint of lukewarm water, stir well and drink often. Repeat the prescription if necessary and it will cure the most obstinate case.

❀

Boil two ounces flaxseed in one quart of water, strain and add two ounces of rock candy, one-half pint of honey, juice of three lemons; mix and let all boil well, let cool and bottle. Take one cupful on going to bed, one-half cupful before meals, the hotter you drink it the better.

For a cough take 1/2 pint vinegar; 1/2 pint rum; 1/4 lb. sugar candy; 6 heads garlic; 1/2 teacup honey. To be simmered down to half the quantity. A tablespoonful 3 times a day.

❀

A bottle of camphorated oil and some absorbent cotton should be kept in the medicine chest of every household. No remedy for coughs will more quickly afford relief than absorbent cotton soaked in the oil and laid on the chest of the sufferer.

❀

To make flaxseed lemonade (good for colds), pour one quart boiling water over four tablespoonfuls of flaxseed. Steep—not boil—three hours; cover closely while steeping; then strain, sweeten to taste, and add the juice of two lemons, putting in more water if too thick to be agreeable.

❀

Cut a turnip in thin slices removing the rind. Cut each slice in five pieces and place in a dish. Cover with brown sugar for 24 hours to form a syrup. Drain juice off and take for a cough or tickle in throat.

❀

Take 2 tablespoonfuls of black currant jam and crush it in a large cup until all the juice comes out. Add 2 teaspoonfuls of sugar and fill the cup with boiling water. Let this sit until cool enough to drink. While drinking this, place feet and ankles in pan of really hot water, as hot as you can stand, into which has been stirred 1 teaspoonful of dry mustard. This was done seated beside the kitchen stove. Go to bed and keep warm for an hour or so—if this is during the day—and the cough or cold will soon disappear. Repeat the drink if necessary.

❀

For sore throat boil 1 pint of vinegar and 1 oz. of myrrh for 1/2 an hour. Pour into a basin which fits the large end of a funnel and inhale from small end. Renew every 1/4 hour till a cure is effected.

❀

When the voice is lost, as is sometimes the case from the effects of cold, a simple pleasant remedy is furnished by beating up the white of one egg, adding to it the juice of one lemon, and sweetening with white sugar to taste. Take a teaspoonful from time to time. It has been known effectually to cure the ailment.

Malarial Fevers

Cold baths, a yarrow and milk plaster applied to the wrists, camomile flowers, hartshorn, lemon, laudanum pills, Peruvian Bark.

❀

Eat one raw lemon with a little salt three times a day and take some good laxative. This keeps the stomach, liver and bowels in good condition.

❀

Give a cathartic and place either onion, garlic or mustard poultices to the feet and apply equal parts of vinegar and water to the head.

❀

For remittent fever, wrap the child in wet cloths until it sweats, then wash in warm water during the fever. Put cloths wrung out of cold water to the head if it is hot and change frequently.

Pneumonia

Cloths wrung out of cold water laid over the chest and renewed every ten minutes, or hot fomentations applied to the chest, well regulated diet, and some good active stimulant. A good dose of castor oil or citrate of magnesia is very beneficial. A flaxseed poultice, half an inch thick placed entirely around the chest is highly recommended. Keep the room at an even temperature.

❀

Take 6 to 10 onions, according to size; chop fine; then add about same quantity of rye meal and enough vinegar to make a thick paste. In the meantime stir it thoroughly, letting it simmer five or ten minutes. Put it in a cotton bag large enough to cover the lungs and apply to the chest as hot as patient can bear. In about ten minutes apply another and thus continue by reheating the poultices, and in a few hours the patient will be out of danger. While it is a simple remedy it has never failed to cure this fatal malady. Usually three or four applications will be sufficient, but continue until perspiration starts.

suffering.

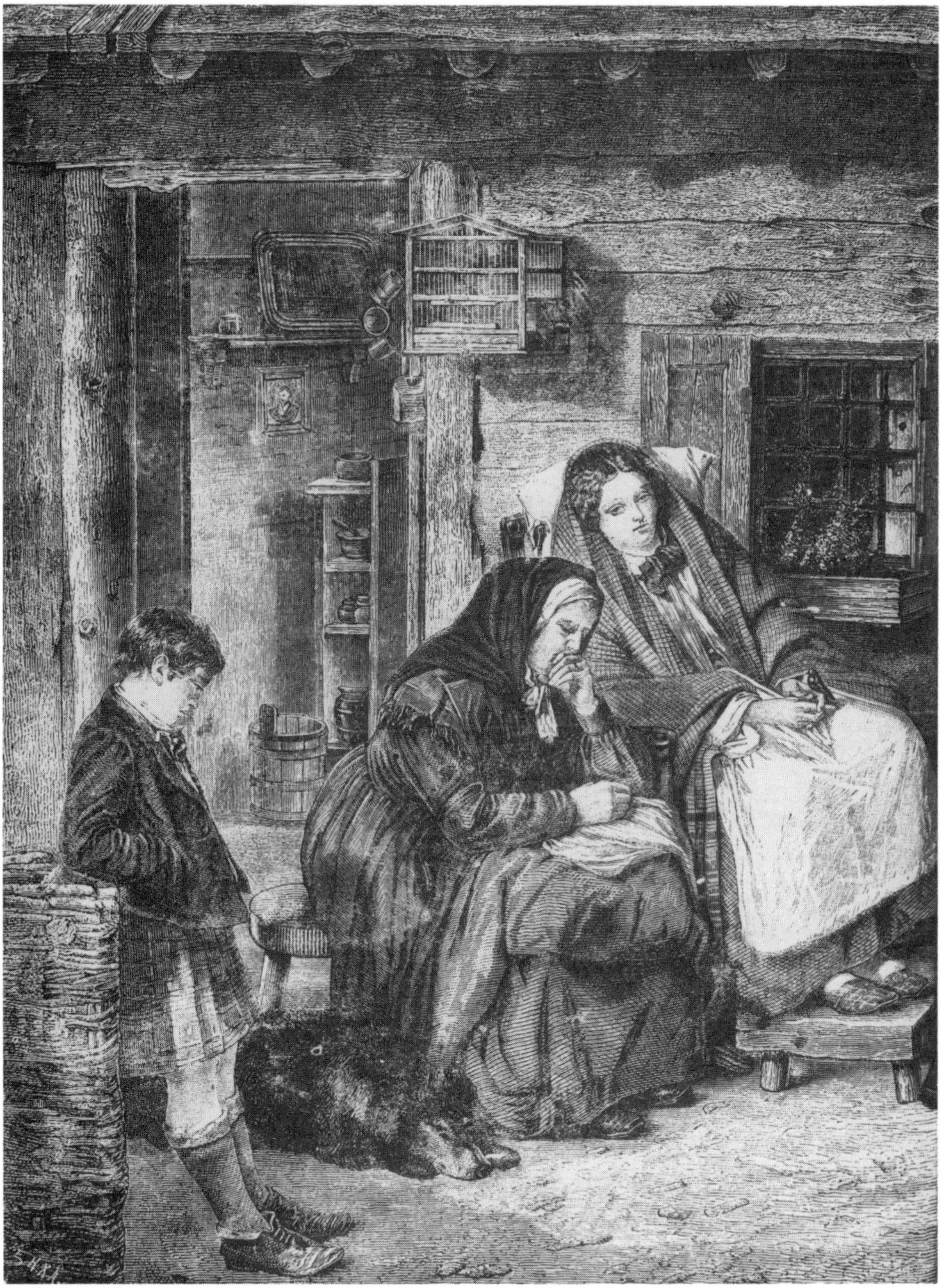

In the Backwoods of Canada, *Canadian Illustrated News*, February 5, 1870

Spasmodic Croup

Probably nine children out of ten who die of croup might be saved by the timely application of roasted onions, mashed and laid upon a napkin, and a small quantity of goose oil, sweet oil, or even lard, put on and applied as hot as can be borne comfortably to the throat and upper part of the chest, and to the feet and hands.

❀

It is claimed that alum and sugar will cure croup in one minute, by shaving or grating off 1 teaspoonful of the alum and mixing it with twice as much sugar, and giving it at once, the relief being almost instantaneous. Half these amounts may be repeated once or twice, 1/2 hour apart, if the relief is not permanent.

❀

Grate a raw onion, squeeze out the juice and add half as much castor oil as you have of the juice. Keep in a bottle well corked, shake before using, and give a teaspoonful every two or three hours.

❀

Goose oil and urine, equal quantities. Take from a tea to a tablespoon of the mixture, according to the age of the child. Repeat the dose every 15 minutes, if the child does not vomit in that time.

❀

Whenever children are threatened with an attack of croup, direct a plaster covered with dry Scotch snuff varying to the age of the patient, to be applied across the top of the thorax and retained there till all the symptoms disappear. The remedy is found to be always effectual when applied in the first and second stages of the malady.

❀

For children who have a tendency to croup, or throat difficulties, get a piece of chamois skin, make it like a little bib, cut out the neck and sew on tapes to tie it on; then melt together some tallow and pine pitch, rub some of this in the chamois, and let the child wear it all the time. Renew this with the mixture occasionally.

❀

For an instantaneous emetic for croup take two teaspoonfuls of mustard mixed in 3 or 4 tablespoonfuls of warm water. This relieves at once by causing vomiting. A teaspoonful of lard warmed and given is also said to serve the same purpose. Either may be repeated if necessary.

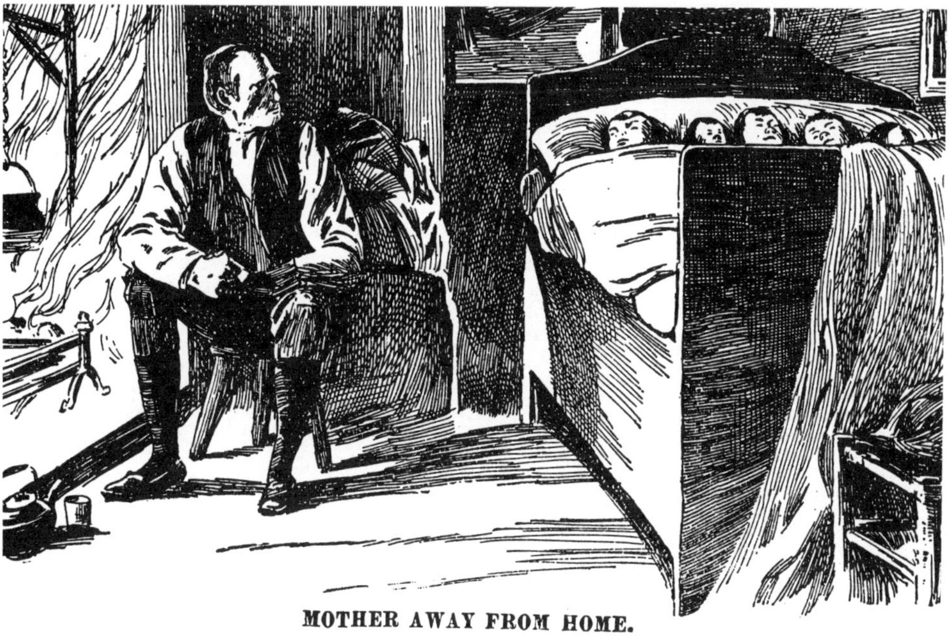

MOTHER AWAY FROM HOME.

Many consider a plaster made of snuff and lard the best application for croup. A teaspoonful of snuff should be mixed with a little lard, spread upon a cloth, and applied to the throat and chest.

❀

Give 5 or 6 drops of lamp oil (kerosene oil) on a lump of sugar. Repeat if necessary. Also apply hot or cold applications externally.

❀

Give some warm melted butter. About a tablespoonful may be given.

❀

If the child is very young apply a poultice of hops boiled in water. During the day when it seems better give a tea made of horseradish and vinegar.

❀

A strip of flannel or a napkin folded lengthwise and dipped in hot water and wrung out and then applied around the neck of a child that has the croup, will often bring instant relief. Apply every five minutes.

❀

Hardly too much can be said in favour of onions as a remedy for coughs and colds; especially for children, they are invaluable. They may be cooked, and eaten at meal time, or, what is better, eaten raw with a little salt, or stirred up in vinegar. A syrup made of them has saved many a child from an attack of croup or lung fever, and where these diseases were fully settled, it has gone far toward a speedy cure. To prepare the syrup, slice an onion in a tin basin, pour upon it half a teacupful of molasses, or, what is better, honey; add a bit of butter as large as a small chestnut; set the dish in the oven, and simmer slowly for an hour. Leave one of the oven doors open, so it will not be too hot. Onions are one of the most nutritious and wholesome of vegetables, and were it not for the shocking odour they leave upon the breath, we should advise everybody to eat them daily. As it is, we can only recommend them in cases of necessity.

❀

Cover the throat and chest with lard and salt paste, adding to it a sprinkling of mustard.

❀

During the paroxysm, dashing cold water in the face is a common remedy. To terminate the spasm and prevent its return, give teaspoonful doses of powdered alum.

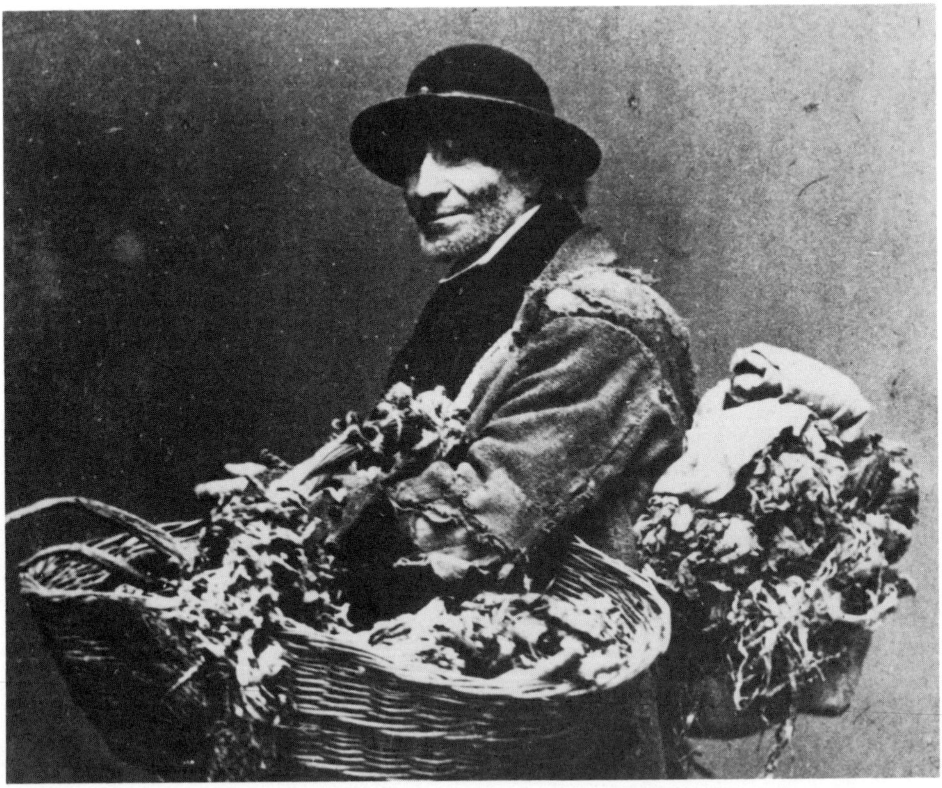

The Herb Doctor c. 1859, Notman Photographic Archives, Montreal

Ear, Nose, Throat and Eyes

Sore Mouth ~ Cankers and Ulcers

Burn a corn cob and apply the ashes two or three times a day for cankers.

❀

Sage tea, honey and borax makes a fine wash for sore mouth and is also a good gargle for sore throat.

❀

Take the scrapings of blackberry root, a few sumach berries, a little saffron, a little sage and some gold thread. Put with these a little alum, some vinegar and honey; simmer this on hot ashes with a little water. Wet the mouth often. It seldom fails to cure.

❀

Boil 1 ounce of white oak bark in a pint of water; strain, and add 1 scruple of alum. Apply several times a day with a soft sponge.

❀

Wash the sore mouth with the juice of ripe tomatoes.

❀

As a gargle for sore mouth use a decoction of witch hazel.

Earache

Digest 2 ozs. bruised garlic in 1 lb. oil of almonds for a week and strain. A drop poured into the ear is effective in temporary deafness.

❀

Make a bag of fine, very soft woollen material or flannel, large enough to cover the affected part. Stitch closely all round the bag leaving one side open. Put into the bag well dried rock salt, enough to fill the bag three parts full, and stitch up. Or, better still, put the salt into a fine cotton bag and put that bag into a good hot oven, until the salt has got very hot right through. Then place a piece of soft material on the bag and lay it on the affected spot. It is a splendid cure for earache.

❀

Take three or four roasted garlics, and while hot mash, and add a tablespoonful of sweet oil and as much honey and laudanum; press out the juice, and drop of this into the ear, warm occasionally. Onion juice is also good in place of garlic.

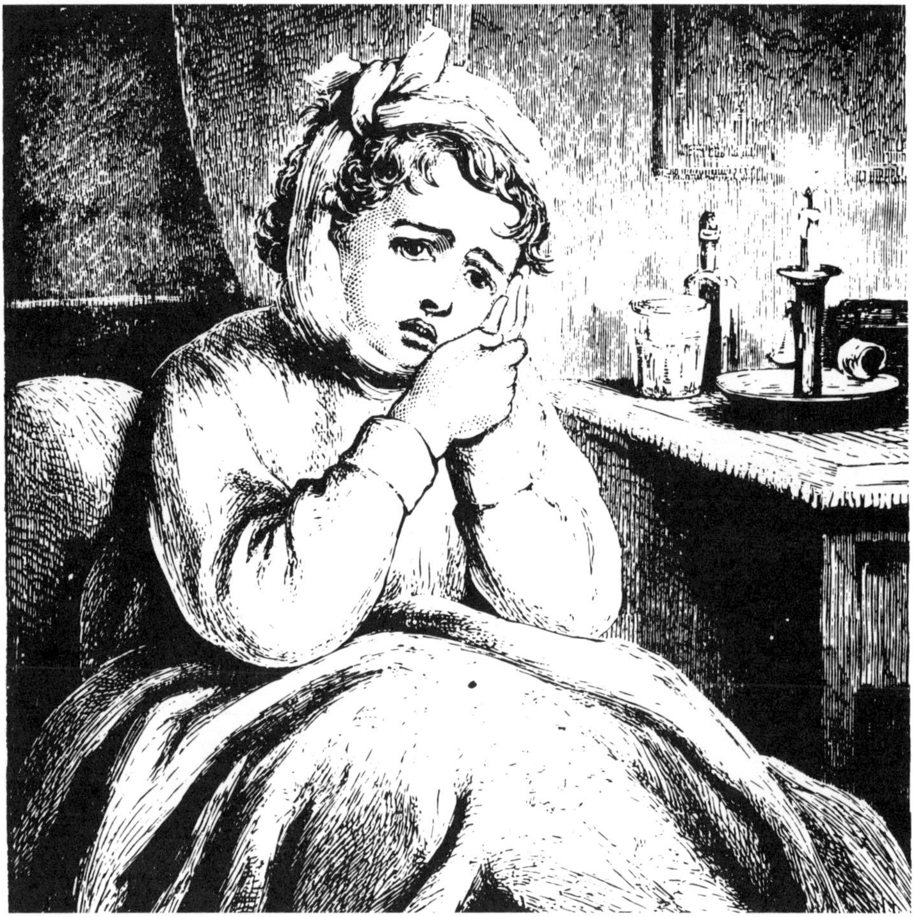

Put the patient's feet in water as hot as can be borne and keep them there for 15 minutes. Put a drop of slightly warmed sweet oil into the ear and put the patient to bed. Take a hot flatiron, wrap a wet cloth around it and then a dry one and place it to the ear. This treatment will bring relief almost instantly.

❀

There is scarcely any ache to which children are subject, so bad to bear and difficult to cure, as the earache. but there is a remedy, never known to fail. Take a bit of cotton batting, put upon it a pinch of black pepper, gather it up and tie it, dip in sweet oil, and insert into the ear. Put a flannel bandage over the head to keep it warm. It will give immediate relief.

Take common tea, one drop, hog's lard, one drop, mix and put in the ear, blood warm—three times a week—then wash the whole head with salt and water.

❀

Bathe the feet in warm water, and drop into the ear a few drops of the following: Take equal parts of laudanum, sweet oil and honey, one part also tincture cayenne; mix, and from a warm teaspoon drop into the ear five or six drops, and stop the ear tight with cotton. Repeat every hour or two. If the pain is very great, steam the ear and side of the head over bitter herbs, and apply a hop fomentation, or a poultice made of roasted onions. Give an active purgative.

❀

Apply hot fomentations, or drop into the ear equal parts of laudanum and sweet oil. A pillow of hops or salt heated and applied to the ear will often furnish relief. If an insect gets into the ear, drop in to the ear a few drops of sweet oil. If there is a discharge in the ear, it should be syringed out every day with warm water.

❀

Take a large onion and cut it into slices; put a slice of onion, then a slice (a piece of leaf the size of the onion) of strong tobacco, then a slice of onion again, then tobacco, till the onion is all laid up, then wrap in a wet cloth and cover in hot embers, till the onion is cooked; press out the juice with heavy pressure, and drop into the ear. It gives instant relief.

❀

That bugbear of the nursery, earache, will soon yield to proper treatment. Make a poultice of hops and vinegar and bind it upon the aching member; almost instant relief will follow. One drop of onion juice and two drops of sweet oil should be put into the ear immediately after the poultice is taken off, to prevent a recurrence of the pain.

Weak and Inflamed Eyes

Half fill a bottle with common rock salt; add the best of French brandy till all but full. Shake it, let it settle, and bathe the outside of the eye with a soft linen cloth on going to bed and occasionally through the day.

❀

For sore eyes, make a tea of wild turnip and lobelia, bathe the eyes at bedtime; open and shut them in cold soft water in the morning.

Mix a few bread crumbs with the white of an egg, put it in a bag of white muslin, and apply it to the eye. It is best applied at night or when lying down. After removing the poultice bathe the eye with warm water, using a piece of soft rag, not a sponge.

❀

Mash some hops and poppy heads; boil in water and make a poultice for the eyes. The water from them may be used for an eye wash.

❀

One of the very best remedies for weak or sore eyes is to bathe them 3 or 4 times a day in weak salt water. This is nature's own remedy for the tears are salty, as we all know. Many eye troubles would be avoided if mothers would see that the children used this simple remedy upon the first appearance of weak eyes.

❀

When the eyes become inflamed from any cause, do not rub them at all—such irritation is dangerous—but bathe them in tepid milk and water, keep the bowels open by some gentle medicine and eat little meat. The eyes are very sensitive to the state of the stomach. Avoid the glare of strong light.

❀

To treat a stye upon the eyelid, put a teaspoonful of black tea in a small bag; pour on it enough boiling water to moisten it; then put it on the eye pretty warm. Keep it on all night and in the morning the stye will most likely be gone; if not, a second application is certain to remove it.

❀

Ordinary tea, when cold, makes a valuable eye-water in many cases.

❀

Take rose leaves, the more the better, and put them into a little water; then boil; after this strain it into a bottle and cork tight. You will find this liquid very beneficial in removing redness and weakness from the eyes.

❀

The juice of the root of garden rhubarb, when applied to the eye, has cured bad eyes.

❀

Cut a slice of stale bread as thin as possible; toast both sides well, but don't burn; when cold, lay in cold spring or ice water; put between a piece of old linen and apply, changing when it gets warm.

Bind some steeped tea leaves on the eyes. Also bathe the eyes in weak salt water. Tea leaves contain tannin which is astringent in its action. This causes the blood vessels to contract, less blood comes to the eyes and the inflammation is reduced.

❀

Apply to the eyes a poultice made of pulverized elm bark, stirred in warm milk and water. The wilted leaves of stramonium (jimson) are also good in severe cases to apply over the eyes.

❀

A teaspoonful of brandy to two tablespoonfuls of water makes a serviceable eye-water when a stimulant is wanted.

❀

For inflammation of the edges of the eyes, melt a little fresh butter in a teaspoonful of milk and wash the eyes when they are glued together in the morning. Afterwards apply a wet sponge to them for several minutes and the lids may be opened without pain.

❀

Make a poultice of some finely scraped raw potato and apply to the eyes every night upon going to bed. It is also excellent for inflamed sores of long standing.

❀

Burn alum, and mix it with the white of eggs and put between two cloths and lay it upon the eyes.

❀

Boil three eggs in water and when at the boiling point add 1/2 ounce of sulphate of zinc and allow it to settle. Use the water for inflammation of the eye of horse, cattle or man. For the human eye it should be reduced by adding ten parts of water.

❀

A rubber bag or bladder filled with pounded ice and held to the eye is a good and safe remedy.

Sore Throat

For sore throat, use an ointment made of equal parts of melted mutton tallow and kerosene oil, stirred until cold, to successfully incorporate the oil; apply outwardly and wrap the throat with a soft cotton cloth; woollen cloth heats, and is liable to blister.

A thin slice of raw fat pork dusted with cayenne pepper is by good authority considered the best remedy for a sore throat, and this is the way to apply it, so the greasy strip shall be securely held in place, poulticing the throat from ear to ear and not slipping down on the collar bone, where it can do little good to swollen tonsils, or rolling away from the throat altogether. Cut a strip of flannel three and one-half inches wide and long enough to pass under the chin and tie on top of the head. Halve this strip lengthwise, leaving an uncut five or six inch length in the centre on which to baste the pork. When this has been sprinkled with cayenne and applied to the throat, tie the upper strings snugly on top of the head and the lower ones at the back of the neck.

❀

Gargle frequently with very hot water or steam the patient's throat with the steam from a teakettle. Either herbs, such as golden seal, horehound, etc., or listerine or turpentine may be added to the kettle of water if you have any of them handy.

❀

Very strong sage tea, 1/2 pt; strained honey, common salt, and strong vinegar, of each 2 tablespoons; cayenne pulverized, one rounding teaspoon; steeping the cayenne with the sage, strain, mix, and bottle for use, gargling from 4 to a dozen times daily according to the severity of the case.

❀

Boil for half an hour a handful each of hops, wormwood, sage, boneset, hoarhound, catnip, or at least three of these articles; and let the patient steam his throat over them, as the hot vapour rises. Put some of the same in a coffee pot, with some vinegar added, and let him inhale the vapour into his mouth, throat and lungs, as warm as he can bear. This will give immediate relief.

❀

Take of sage, 2 ozs; linseed, 1 oz; boiling water, 1 pint. Mix. To be used cold in the early stages of inflamed throat.

❀

If you have sore throat try chewing some tea leaves.

❀

Place a piece of brown paper saturated with kerosene oil around the neck and gargle with a solution made of equal parts of salt and alum.

For local treatment of the throat, the simple home-made gargle of vinegar, salt and water is good for a slight attack, but for one more severe, dissolve chlorate of potash in water in the proportion of a teaspoonful of chlorate to a pint of water. Gargle the throat every half hour, using caution about swallowing much of it, as the chlorate is poisonous if taken in large quantities.

❀

A teaspoonful of powdered borax to two tablespoonfuls of honey. Warm in the oven in a small cup or china pot, stirring until it is dissolved. When cool, apply it repeatedly with a camel's hair brush to the throat and roof of mouth; this will soon effect a cure, and enable the patient to swallow.

Tonsillitis

Put hot flaxseed or hop poultices to the throat; change every few minutes and relief will soon follow.

❀

Take 1 tablespoonful of honey, 2 tablespoonfuls of vinegar and enough sage tea to make half a pint. Use as a gargle.

❀

To a pint of water and vinegar add a tablespoonful of salt and a teaspoonful of cayenne and simmer together. Cool, strain, and use as a gargle.

❀

Into a kettle containing 2 quarts of boiling water put either 5 drops of carbolic acid or 3/4 of a teaspoonful of turpentine and steam the patient's throat in the following manner—Attach a piece of hose to the spout of the boiling kettle. If you have no hose, take a tube or roll of paper, put one end over the spout and the other end of the tube or hose in the mouth of the patient and have him inhale the steam. Make the tube as short as possible so that the steam will be as hot as the patient can bear it. The hot steam enters the mouth and relieves the painful and swollen parts.

Toothache

One ounce alcohol, two drams cayenne pepper, one ounce kerosene oil; mix, and let stand twenty-four hours—a sure cure.

❀

Apply powdered alum and salt, equal parts; saturate a piece of cotton with a strong solution of ammonia and apply to the tooth. A poultice of slippery elm bark and cold water sometimes gives relief.

❀

Put a piece of quicklime, as big as a walnut, in a pint of water in a bottle. Clean the teeth with a little of it every morning, rinsing the mouth with clean water afterward. If the teeth are good, it will preserve them and keep away the toothache; if the teeth are gone, it will harden the gums, so that they will masticate crusts and all.

❀

The worst toothache, or neuralgia coming from the teeth, may be speedily ended by the application of a small bit of clean cotton saturated in a strong solution of ammonia to the defective tooth. Sometimes the application causes nervous laughter, but the pain has disappeared.

❀

Horseradish root, bruised and bound upon the face, or other parts where pain is located, has been found very valuable for their relief.

❀

Equal parts of powdered alum and salt, mixed, then wet a bit of cotton, to make the powder adhere, and apply to the hollow of the tooth.

❀

Take an ounce of spirit of camphor, 3 drams of liquor ammonia, 10 drops of essential oil of bergamot. Mix them in a vial for use.

❀

Split a raisin, put a little mustard on the sticky side and apply to the aching tooth or gum. It will draw out all the soreness.

❀

Put 2 drams of camphor into an ounce of oil of turpentine, and let it dissolve, when it will be fit for use.

❀

The worst case of toothache can be cured by chewing a piece of the root of the large field thistle which is commonly known as the "bull" thistle;

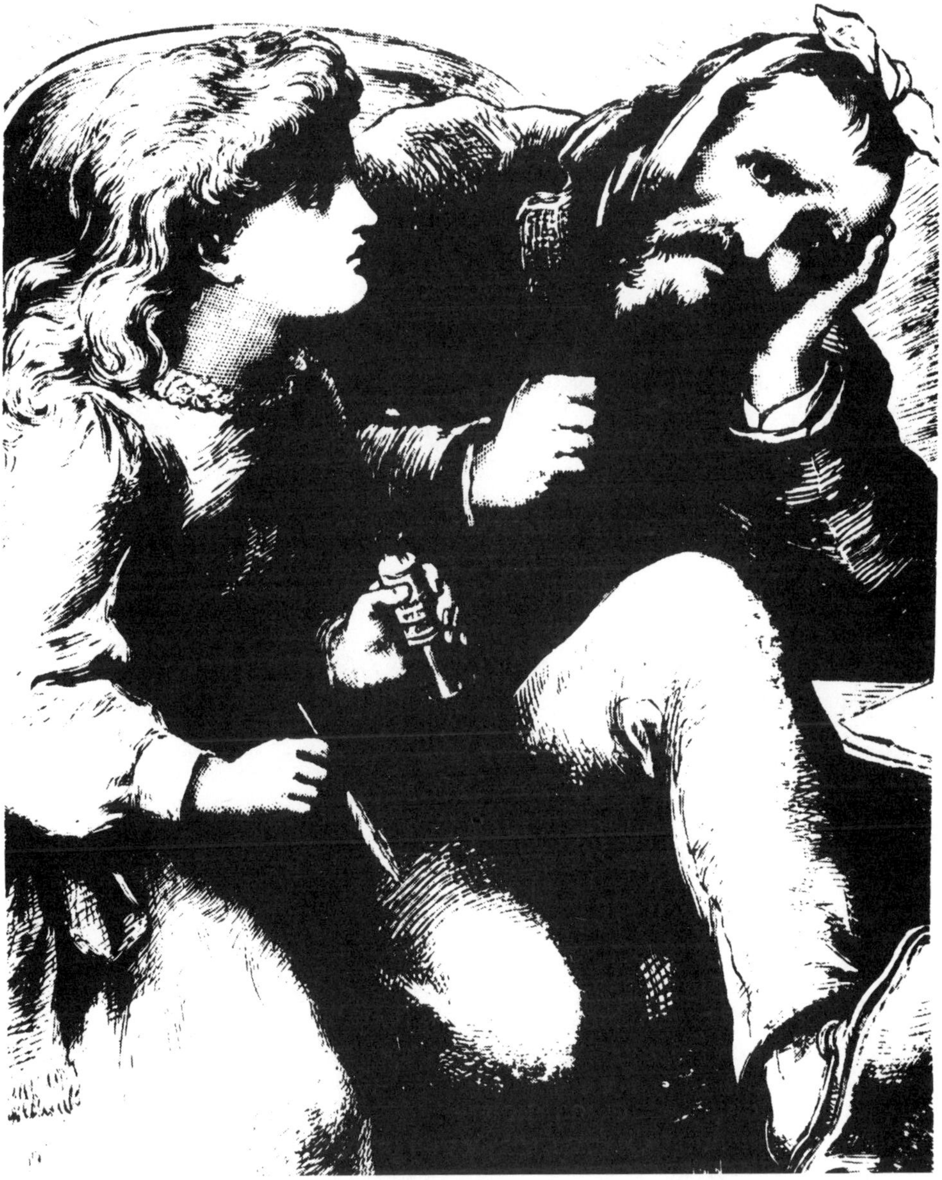

and, by drinking a tea and applying a poultice made from its leaves you can permanently cure the worst case of neuralgia that ever existed.

❀

If the toothache comes from decayed teeth it may be relieved by holding rum, brandy, whisky or diluted tincture of cayenne in the mouth. It will also help to apply laudanum or a mustard plaster externally.

Put in to the tooth a pill made of camphor gum and opium. Stop up the ear with cotton or wool as tight as you can on the side on which the aching tooth is situated. This seldom fails to cure in the course of a day or night.

❀

Steep a piece of coarse brown paper in cold vinegar, then grate ginger on it, and apply to the side of the face affected; the application to be made at bedtime and kept on during the whole of the night.

❀

To half an ounce of chloroform add half a dram each of oil of cinnamon, oil of cloves and creosote and with a little piece of cotton bathe the gums on both sides of the tooth and, if there is a cavity, insert some of the cotton which has been wet with the mixture.

❀

A towel folded several times and quickly wrung out of hot water and applied over the face will relieve, and many times cure, toothache and neuralgia.

❀

Mix gun powder and tallow and put it in the cavity.

Other Ailments and Treatments

Syrups, Herbs & Blood Purifiers

The safest and quickest prescription for clearing the blood is to eat a raw onion, finely minced, at breakfast; the whole of a common sized onion is enough, and a dose of charcoal or ground coffee, and brushing the teeth, will deodorize the breath. The onion can be taken with salt and vinegar as a salad.

❀

Sulphur and molasses with a little cream of tartar added is a fine blood remedy. Take three days and skip three days. The dose is a teaspoonful. Cream of tartar is a diuretic and acts on the kidneys and it is also a laxative and aids in casting off the impurities. Sulphur is an alterative and a laxative and thus cleanses the blood.

❀

To 1 quart of hard cider add 1 ounce of yellow dock root and 1/2 ounce of horseradish. Take a wineglassful 4 times a day. This is one of the best blood purifiers known and saves you the dollar you would otherwise pay the druggist for patent medicine as it can be made at home.

❀

Burdock is a good blood remedy. It may be used as a decoction or a syrup. Take 1/2 pint three times a day. Burdock is better when in combination with other remedies.

Haemorrhoids/Piles

Mix one tablespoon of sulphur with half a pint of milk, to be taken every day until favourable symptoms appear, and then occasionally, as the case may require. The above is a cheap, simple, and most infallible cure for that most painful and unpleasant disorder. It is equally useful as a preventive.

❀

Take sweet alder, the inner bark, and white oak bark, simmer it in sweet cream, the juice of camomile pounded and pressed out, and mix a tablespoonful of this with a gill of the above, and use it night and morning constantly.

Take half an ounce of cut tobacco, place it on a pan over the fire and burn it to ashes (don't let it blaze), then mix it with lard, one teacupful, one tablespoonful of turpentine, melt together—anoint three or four times a day.

❀

Keep the bowels well opened by a mild aperient such as castor oil, or senna tea, and apply to the part the following ointment: hemlock bark finely powdered—1 oz., fresh lard—6 ozs. Mix and apply.

❀

Take, say a teacupful of hog's lard (more or less), put in a flat tin or pewter dish, and take two bars of lead, flattened a little, and rub the lard with flat ends, and between them till it becomes black or a dark lead colour. Then burn equal parts of cavendish tobacco and old shoe-leather in an iron vessel till charred; powder these and mix into the lard till it becomes a thick ointment. Use once or twice a day as an ointment for the piles. A never failing cure.

❀

Take oyster shells, wash and burn them, then finely pulverize and rub up with fresh lard; anoint with this, and take internally sulphur one ounce, mixed with three ounces of pulverized rosin; take night and morning what will lay on a five cent piece. Take every day for the first week, then every three or four days, until well, continuing the ointment.

❀

Make an ointment by taking 1 tablespoonful of fresh butter and 2 teaspoonfuls of turpentine, adding a little salt. Several times a day apply this ointment either outside or inside the rectum.

❀

Mix 2 ounces of sulphur with 1/2 pound of melted lard and stir until cold. This is one of the finest ointments made for piles, tetter, salt rheum, itch and skin diseases in general.

❀

Cover 2 ounces of fine cut tobacco with spirits and add 1/2 pound of lard and simmer over a slow fire until the tobacco is a little crisp and then strain. This ointment is also valuable for shingles and skin diseases.

❀

Equal parts of chopped raisins, tobacco and lard makes one of the best remedies known for piles.

Make a decoction of witch hazel, apple tree bark and white oak bark, and mix with lard to make a salve. This is very good for piles.

❀

Where there is much pain a hip-bath of fifteen to twenty minutes, if the pain is very severe it will produce relief. Applying a bread and milk poultice four or five times a day is also a good remedy.

❀

For an external application take the inner bark of the white oak tree, boil and strain, and boil again until you obtain 1/2 pint of the extract, very thick; then add 1/2 pint of the oil of the oldest and strongest bacon you can procure; simmer together until a union takes place when cold. Then apply by the finger up the rectum every night until well. Be very strict to abstain from strong and stimulating diet. The above is a sure cure for blind or bleeding piles, in all cases, sooner or later.

❀

For blind or bleeding piles apply an ointment made by taking 1 dram of sulphur and 2 ounces of lard. Rub this mixture between two flat pieces of lead until the ointment is blackened.

❀

Remove the shells from 6 horse chestnuts, or buckeyes; chop them fine, add enough lard to just cover the nuts; and let them stand for an hour near the fire. Strain, and when cool apply the lard or ointment to the parts twice a day. This is a very valuable remedy for piles.

❀

The ingredients are: 2 tablespoonfuls of tar, 8 tablespoonfuls of lard, not heaped. First wash the parts effected with castile soap and water, and then apply the ointment. The ointment should be used once or twice each day.

Insects/Bugs

To prevent gnat and midge bites, sprinkle your stocking with violet powder mixed with a small amount of white pepper. A sprinkling of oil of lavender or oil of geranium is also an excellent cure.

❀

Sometimes hartshorn is applied to the skin in the vicinity of the wound; some people consider a cabbage leaf the best possible application. The fact is, that anything which serves to cool the surface diminishes the irritation and pain.

To one pint of milk add a quarter of a pound of raw sugar, and two ounces of ground pepper; simmer them together eight or ten minutes, and place it about in shallow dishes. The flies attack it greedily, and in a few moments are suffocated. By this method kitchens, etc. may be kept clear of flies all summer, without the danger attending poison.

❀

Scatter a little green sage on the shelves and floor where insects are troublesome, and they will leave the premises.

❀

If a person be stung in the mouth or throat, the swelling which results is apt to be so great as to embarrass the breathing. In such a case the patient should even before the parts are much swollen, employ faithfully gargles of hot water containing a little borax. A popular remedy is a mixture of vinegar and water, which is heated and used as a gargle.

❀

To kill cockroaches, strew the floor for three or four nights with cucumber peel—the cockroaches suck the juice and it poisons them.

❀

A piece of lean raw meat will instantly relieve the sting of a wasp or bee. Soda and vinegar is also an excellent remedy.

❀

For bee stings and bites of insects, take pulverized borax 1 ounce, water 1 1/2 pints. Boil down to 1 pint, and then touch the parts every 2 or 3 hours with swab dipped in the above, as long as there is any itching or irritation.

❀

Insect bites, and even that of a rattlesnake, have passed harmless by stirring enough of common salt into the yolk of an egg to make it sufficiently thin for a plaster, to be kept on the bitten parts.

❀

As a cure for bee and wasp stings, spider bites, etc., apply ammonia or common soda and water. If there is much inflammation and redness, apply a solution of borax and warm water. Apply with a rag saturated with the solution.

Insomnia

Lie with the head to the North, for there is no doubt something in the electrical effects of the earth upon the body when in that position.

❀

Bad sleepers should always rise early and retire early, and they should never take a nap during the day. Sleepless persons should avoid exciting conversation or reading, hard study, or any kind of mental excitement during the evening. When lying in bed, first draw in the breath slowly, letting it out suddenly, then draw it in suddenly and let it pass slowly out a number of times alternately.

❀

There is no fact more clearly established in the physiology of man than this, that the brain expends its energies and itself during the hours of wakefulness and that these are recuperated during sleep. If the recuperation does not equal the expenditure, the brain withers; this is insanity.

❀

For those troubled with sleeplessness from literary labour, or other disturbances of the nervous system, the following is highly recommended—just before retiring, eat two or three small raw onions, with a little bread, lightly spread with fresh butter, which will produce the desired effect, saving the stupefying action of drugs.

❀

A cold bath, or a sponge bath and rubbing or a good run, or a rapid walk in the open air, or going up or down stairs a few times just before retiring, will aid in equalizing circulation and promoting sleep. These rules are simple and easy of application, in castle or cabin.

❀

Wet half a towel, apply it to the back of the neck, pressing it upward to the base of the brain, and fasten the dry half of the towel over so as to prevent the too rapid evaporation. The effect is prompt, cooling the brain and inducing calmer, sweeter sleep than any narcotic. Warm water may be used though most persons prefer cold. To those suffering from over excitement of the brain, whether the result of brain work or pressing anxiety, this simple remedy is an especial boon.

Poisons ~ Antidotes

When it becomes known that a poison has been swallowed, stir salt and ground mustard, of each a heaping teaspoon, into a glass of water, and have it drunk immediately. It is the quickest emetic known.

❀

It is said that raw eggs and milk are a sure remedy for poison of any kind taken into the stomach. This is information that may do a deal of good if remembered and cannot possibly be productive of any harm.

❀

For rattlesnake bite drink whisky until drunkenness and stupor are produced, which goes to show that the bite of the *Devil's tea* is worse than the bite of a rattlesnake.

❀

Quickly mix a couple of ounces of powdered chalk or magnesia with a pint of milk and swallow the whole at one draught. Then run the finger down the throat and move it gently from side to side. This will induce vomiting; after which drink freely of warm milk and water and repeat the vomiting.

❀

When the mucous membrane of the mouth is much inflamed or destroyed, give raw eggs, flour stirred in water, flaxseed tea, arrowroot, or any soothing drink. Stimulation can be applied by means of hot water bottles or bags to the feet and over the heart, and by rubbing the extremities. Alcoholic stimulant should be administered very cautiously.

❀

To neutralize any poisonous mineral or vegetable, taken intentionally or by accident, swallow 2 gills (1/2 pt.) of sweet oil; for a strong constitution more oil.

❀

If a person swallows any poison whatever, or has fallen into convulsions from having overloaded the stomach, an instantaneous remedy, more efficient and applicable in a number of cases than any half-a-dozen medicines we can now think of, is a heaping teaspoonful of salt and as much ground mustard, stirred rapidly in a teacup of water, warm or cold, and swallowed instantly. It is scarcely down before it begins to come up, bringing with it remaining contents of the stomach; and lest there be any remnant of poison, however small, let the white of an egg, or a teacup of strong coffee, be swallowed as soon as the stomach is quiet; because these very common articles nullify a larger number of virulent poisons than any medicines in the shops.

❀

Some propose as an antidote for every case of poisoning, half a pint of bland oil, as sweet oil, fresh butter melted to oil, etc., to be drunk at once, for an adult.

Poultices

Poultices should be applied soft and moist but not thin enough to run over the surrounding parts. They are usually applied warm and renewed before they become dry or cool. Various poultices are used for the purpose of scattering tumours, stimulating, checking mortification, lessening inflammation, hastening the formation of pus or drawing poison from wounds.

❀

Corn Meal Poultice - This poultice is made by cooking corn meal in hot water until it sticks together. Apply to the seat of the pain as hot as it can be borne.

❀

Pork/Onion Poultice - Take raw salt pork and about the same bulk in boiled onions, and chop together thoroughly fine in a wooden bowl and apply warm and bind on about half an inch thick on the injured or wounded parts.

❀

Soothing Poultices - Poultices of bread and milk, flaxseed, corn meal or slippery elm are used where a soothing effect is desired as they retain heat and moisture a long time. The bread and milk and flaxseed poultices are best for boils, felons and abscesses when they are forming. After the matter begins to discharge the slippery elm poultice should be used. Slippery elm is also best for deep ulcers and carbuncles.

❀

Mullein Poultice - Boil mullein leaves in water and with this make a thin mush with corn meal and add just a little vinegar.

❀

Flaxseed Poultice - While water is boiling, add flaxseed to it very slowly until it becomes as thick as porridge. Continue the heat with constant stirring for 10 minutes, then spread on cotton and cover with gauze or cheese cloth which makes the covering next to the skin. Cover the whole with silk or flannel to retain the heat and, if necessary, bandage snugly to keep it from slipping. Renew when cool.

❀

Spice Poultice - Mix equal parts of ground cinnamon, cloves, all-spice and ginger and if you wish to have it very strong, you can add 1/4 part of cayenne pepper. Place this in a flannel bag and spread evenly and wet with alcohol or whisky before applying. This will last for a long time by rewetting. It is fine for pains in the abdomen.

❀

Clay Poultice - Take the stratum of clay used for making the best red brick, which lies immediately below the soil. Dry in the sun so it can be put through a sieve; keep in air-tight jars; mix with hot water until of the consistency of putty, and apply warm, with a knife, over the tumour, half an inch thick; cover with light brown paper, then bandage with a good strong bandage, and keep it on 24 to 48 hours. This has caused some wonderful cures. It is also good for some forms of rheumatism, dropsy and poisoned wounds.

❀

Bran Poultice - When a light but thick poultice is required, bran should be boiled in water and placed in a bag and tied tightly. Press out the surplus water and apply to the parts. Cover well as it cools quickly. Instead of bran, hops can be used and applied in the same way.

❀

Cranberry Poultice - Bruise the desired quantity of cranberries and apply to the throat for quinsy and to swollen glands in scarlet fever and other diseases. Also fine for erysipelas. It gives relief in a few hours.

❀

Robinson's Salve or Poultice, for Sores, Inflammation, etc.—Scrape plenty of raw potatoes and thicken it with finely pulverized charcoal. Apply freely to the sore, or inflamed part, and renew as often as it becomes dry, or once in 3 or 4 hours.

❀

Mustard Poultice - For a mustard poultice, a sufficient quantity of powdered mustard should be taken to make a thin paste the required size. This should be mixed with boiling water, with a small quantity of vinegar added, if a very strong poultice is required, and spread on brown paper, with a piece of thin muslin over it. A mustard poultice should generally be kept on from ten to twenty minutes, but some skins will bear it much

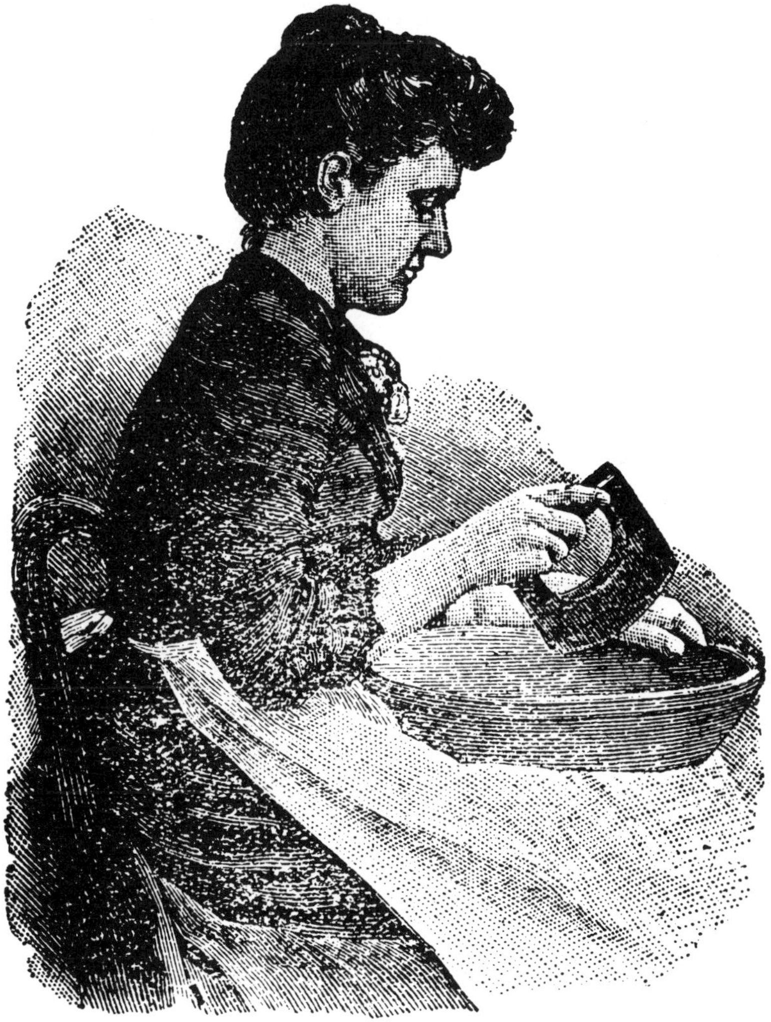

MAKING A PORK AND ONION POULTICE.

longer than others. If the skin is very irritable afterwards, a little flour should be sprinkled over it. This will remove the burning sensation.

Linseed Poultice - Put the linseed into a basin and pour over enough boiling water to make it into a stiff paste. Always mix with a warm spoon or knife. Spread the linseed on one half of a piece of muslin, and cover over with the other half of the muslin. Apply as hot as possible.

Charcoal Poultice - The charcoal may either be mixed with the ingredients of the poultice or sprinkled over the part and covered with simple poultice, or the following receipt may be used. Take of:- Wood charcoal (powder), 1 tablespoonful; Bread, 3 or 4 slices; Flaxseed meal, 3 tablespoonfuls; Boiling water, 1 tumblerful. Mix. A useful application to offensive wounds and sores.

❀

Onion Poultice - For boils, inflammation of the bowels, etc.—A poultice of roasted onions applied to boils, tumours, etc., hastens suppuration, and are often applied as "drafts" to the feet, and are applied in excessive fevers, by mashing or pounding onions and placing them under the arms and upon the bowels or other parts swollen from extensive inflammation (to be changed often), and they are very valuable indeed.

❀

Yeast Poultice - Applicable to sores and indolent ulcers. Made by taking 5 ounces of yeast and a pound of flour (or in that proportion), and adding to water at blood heat, so as to form a tolerably stiff dough; set in a warm place (but not so as to scald) until it begins to ferment or to "rise," and apply like any poultice.

❀

Irish moss has been suggested as a substitute for flaxseed meal in poultices. It is said to make a superior poultice, as it keeps moist about eighteen hours, does not slip, is inodorous, and neither ferments easily nor soils the bed clothes or linen of the patient.

❀

For ulcerated sores and swellings, use 1 lb. garden carrots, boiled and bruised, 1 oz. flour and 1/2 oz. butter. Mix and make into a poultice.

❀

Bread and Milk Poultice - Pour boiling milk on the crumbs of stale wheat bread in a basin. Stir with a back of a spoon until the mass is brought to the thickness and consistency of mush. Spread upon a piece of cloth folded several times and a little larger than the surface intended to be covered. This is an excellent poultice, subject to the only disadvantage of souring quickly. It must therefore be frequently changed.

Rheumatism/Arthritis

For muscular rheumatism keep the affected parts warm and bathe two or three times a day with arnica. Rub it in with a coarse flannel, stimulating the muscles by thorough rubbing. A hot bath at bedtime to induce free perspiration. A rheumatic person should wear woollen garments next to the skin and also sleep in warm blankets during the cold season of the year. Take a good dose of rhubarb at bedtime.

❀

For painful joints apply equal parts of whisky and vinegar.

❀

To one quart of alcohol add two tablespoonfuls of pulverized potash and a lump of gum camphor the size of an egg. Use as a liniment.

❀

Take half a pint of horseradish root, half a pint of mustard seed, half a tablespoonful of cayenne; put all in one quart of brandy. Dose, one tablespoonful four times a day in hemlock tea—for chronic rheumatism.

❀

To 1 pint of vinegar add 1/8 pint of turpentine and into this break an egg, shell and all. Rub on the parts several times a day.

❀

Take 1 oz. ginger; 1 oz black pepper; 1 oz mustard; 1 oz. sulphur; 2 ozs. honey; and 1 quart beer or a bottle of Port wine. Take 1 tablespoonful.

❀

Chronic rheumatism has been cured in twenty-four hours, after two years' suffering, by using alcohol, spirits of turpentine, sweet spirits of nitre, and oil of juniper, equal parts of each; mix; rub well into the parts, and take ten drops at bedtime in water.

❀

Kerosene oil, 3 ozs; skunk's oil, 1 oz; mix, and shake when applied. Put it on quite freely, and heat it by the stove, or by means of a hot shovel.

❀

Take rum, 1 pt; neats-foot oil, 1/2 pt; or if the joint is stiff, skunk's oil instead of the other spirits of turpentine, 1 gill; and simmer them together, and bottle for use, rubbing it in thoroughly 3 times daily.

Take cucumbers, when full grown, and put them into a pot with a little salt; then put the pot over a slow fire, where it should remain for about an hour; then take the cucumbers and press them, the juice from which must be put into bottles, corked up tight, and placed in the cellar, where they should remain for about a week; then wet a flannel rag with the liquid, and apply it to the parts affected.

❀

Take 1 lb. of epsom salts and add 1 quart of boiling water and the juice of 5 lemons. Add 1 tablespoonful cream of tartar then slice 1 lemon and add sufficient water to make 2 quarts. Take largest dose first, about 3 wineglassfuls, then 1 wineglassful to be taken before bed time.

❀

To a pint of sweet oil add an ounce of pulverized saltpetre and you have a cheap but very effective application for inflammatory rheumatism.

❀

Steep, but not boil, two teaspoonfuls of cayenne pepper in a teacupful of good vinegar, strain, and bottle for use. This will cause heat and is fine for rheumatism.

❀

Chronic rheumatism has been cured by taking the bark of a bearing crab-apple tree, and putting a sufficient amount of it into whisky to make it very strong, then taking a wineglass three times daily, until a gallon was used.

❀

For rheumatism take 4 ounces each of spirits of turpentine and linseed oil add 2 ounces each of iodine and aqua ammonia; mix, shake, and apply as needed.

❀

For stiffened joints take of the bark of white oak and sweet apple trees equal parts. Boil them down to a thick substance and then add the same quantity of goose grease or oil and simmer together. Rub it on the affected parts, warm.

❀

A very simple remedy for rheumatism of the extremities, and one that very often gives great relief is, to take a large piece of thick flannel, sprinkle it well with finely pulverized sulphur, and then bind snugly about the limb, with the sulphur next to the skin.

Take oil of linseed, oil of cedar, and oil of amber, of each one ounce; gum camphor, half ounce; dissolve in half an ounce of sweet oil, by rubbing in a mortar, first adding to the camphor a few drops of alcohol, so as to powder it; spirits of turpentine and laudanum, of each half an ounce. Mix, shake well, and apply, and rub in well. One of the best rheumatic liniments known.

❀

One-quarter small teaspoonful Canadian balsam. Take three times a day after meals, a little water taken afterwards, and also rub the affected part twice a day with coal oil until a warm glow is felt.

❀

Cayenne pepper, 2 teaspoonfuls, steeped in 1 teacup of good vinegar, and the parts affected to be bathed with it. After steeping (not to boil), strain and bottle for use. It will cause considerable heat of the surface, and would, even, if a pint of vinegar were used. Apply 2 or 3 times daily, and if limb is very painful, wet cloths in the mixture and wrap around it, as long as it can be borne.

❀

For arthritis take 2 teaspoonfuls alfalfa seed; 3 and 1/2 cups water. Boil for 20 minutes, then let stand for 10 minutes. Strain into three cups and take 3 times daily at 10 A.M., 3 P.M. and 7 P.M.

❀

Twenty drops solution of potash 3 times a day in a wineglass of water.

❀

An excellent liniment for rheumatism, sprains & bruises is to take one ounce spirits of ammonia, one ounce spirits of turpentine, one ounce tincture of opium, one pint rain water, add a little soap. Shake well before using. Bathe affected part well with hot water before applying.

❀

Half ounce of strongest camphorated spirit, one ounce spirits of turpentine, one raw egg, half pint best vinegar. Well mix the whole, and keep it closely corked. To be rubbed in three or four times a day. For rheumatism in the head, or face-ache, rub all over the back of the head and neck, as well as the part which is the immediate seat of pain.

❀

Take about half a pint of angle-worms (usually known as fish-worms), put them in a glass bottle, add one ounce of oil of sassafras and spirits of turpentine, and two tablespoonfuls of salt, and let stand in the sun two or three days, or till they are dissolved; or if there is no sun, dissolve by gentle heat near the fire; then strain through flannel to exclude the dirt, and bottle for use. This liniment, freely used twice a day, and persevered in, will overcome the stiffness of any joint, where it is possible to do so. As an auxiliary, the joint should be steamed over hot bitter herbs once a day, or a hot fomentation of bitter herbs applied and bound on at night, such as hops, tansy, catnip, horehound, smart-weed, jimson leaves, and the like. A poultice of wheat bran, made with a decoction of bitter herbs, and applied hot, is also very good, and should be used occasionally at night.

❀

As a liniment for rheumatism 2 oz. wintergreen; 2 oz. camphor gum; 2 oz. gasoline.

❀

The celery should be cut into bits, boiled in water until soft, and the water drunk by the patient. Put new milk, with a little flour and nutmeg, in a saucepan, with boiled celery, serve with pieces of toast, eat it with potatoes, and the painful ailment will soon yield.

❀

For rheumatic pains or the lumbago dissolve as much salt in water as will make it swim an egg, rub it with your hand on the part affected before a fire, for 15 or 20 minutes, just before going to bed.

❀

Bathe the part affected in water in which potatoes with their skins on have been boiled, as hot as can be borne, just before going to bed. By the next morning the pain will be much relieved, if not removed. One application of this simple remedy has cured the most obstinate rheumatic pains.

Salves

For sore nipples, apply a plaster of balsam fir, when the child has done sucking.

❀

Salve for Fever Sores, Abscesses, Broken Breasts, etc.—Thoroughly steep tobacco, 1/2 oz., in soft water 1 pt., straining out from the tobacco and boiling down to 1 gill; then have melted, lard, rosin, and beeswax, of each 1/2 oz. simmering to a thick salve, then stirring in 1 gill of old rum, and, if necessary, continuing the simmering a little longer. To be used as other salves.

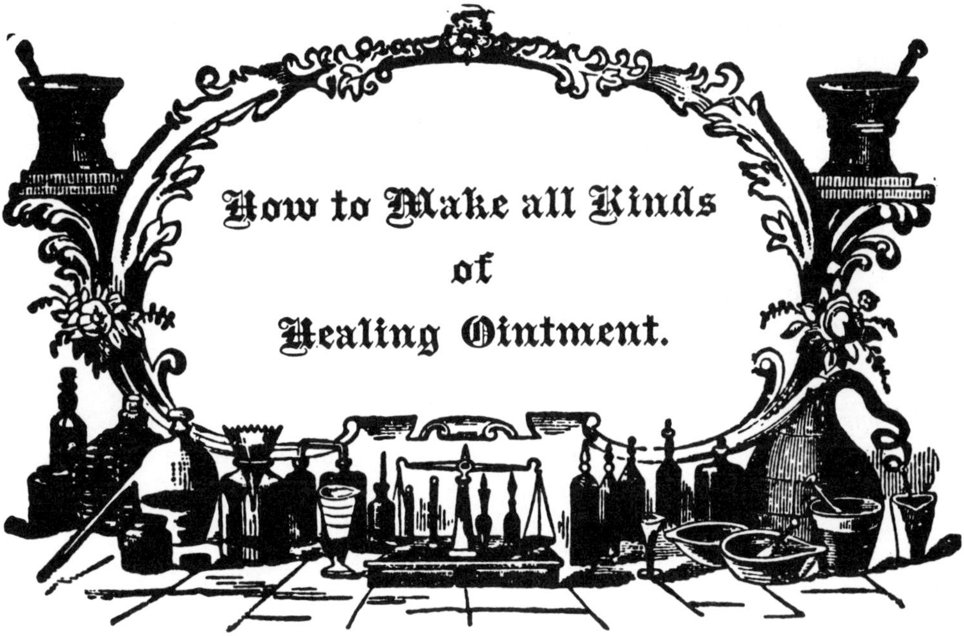

HOW TO MAKE ALL KINDS OF OINTMENT.

Common Ointment - Take yellow wax, 1 oz; olive oil, 4 ozs; lard, 1 oz. Mix. A soothing salve.

❀

Grandmother's Salve for Everything - Two pounds of resin and half a teacup of mutton tallow after it is hard, half as much beeswax, and half an ounce of camphor gum; put all together into an old kettle, and let it dissolve and just come to a boil, stirring with a stick; then take half a pail of warm water, just the chill off, pour it in and stir carefully until you can get your hands around it. Two persons must each take half and pull like candy until quite white and brittle; put a little grease on your hands to prevent sticking, and keep them wet all the time. Wet the table, roll out the salve, and cut it with a knife. Keep it in a cool place.

❀

Sumach Ointment - The following has cured some very severe cases of fever sore and is good for cuts and bruises in man or beast. Take a quantity of the bark of sumach root and boil for two hours; strain and add fresh lard to the liquid, then boil down until the water is all out; anoint the sore three times a day.

Toad Ointment - For sprains, strains, lame-back, rheumatism, caked breasts, etc.

Good sized live toads, 4 in number; put into boiling water and cook very soft; then take them out and boil the water down to 1/2 pint, and add fresh churned, unsalted butter, 1 lb., and simmer together; at the last add tincture of arnica, 2 ozs. This was obtained from an old Physician, who thought more of it than of any other prescription in his possession. Some persons might think it hard on toads, but you could not kill them quicker in any other way.

❀

Magnetic Ointment for Man and Beast - 1 pound elder bark; 1 pound spikenard; 1 pound yellow dock root. Boil 2 gallons of water down to 1, then press the strength out of the roots and boil the liquid down to 1/2 gallon; add 8 pounds of the best resin, 1 pound of beeswax, and tallow enough to soften. Roll in rolls, and apply by warming and spreading on linen.

❀

Take fresh hog dung and lard and mix it, and put it right on the effected part.

❀

Ointment - Sweet clover (grown in gardens) stewed in lard; then add beeswax and white pine turpentine, equal parts, to form an ointment, is highly recommended.

❀

Salve or Plaster for Chaps, Cracks, etc. - Rosin, 10 ozs; mutton tallow, 2 ozs; beeswax, 1 oz. Simmer together and work as shoemakers do their wax, and make it into convenient rolls. Spread on slips of cloth to suit the place, and apply as hot as the flesh will bear it—it will need no tying. If too stiff in very cold weather use a little more tallow and beeswax, or a little less rosin.

❀

Salve for Fever Sores, Cuts, etc. - Spirits of turpentine and honey, of each 1/2 pint, simmered over a slow fire until they unite by stirring; then set aside to cool until you can put in the yolk of an egg without its being cooked by the heat; stir it in and return it to the fire, adding camphor gum 1/4 oz., simmer and stir until well mixed.

Salve for Inflamed Wounds - Lard, 8 ozs., melted 3 or 4 times, and cooled each time in cold water (vaseline or cosmoline is now used without the purification, and will do as well, and possibly better); then stew in it 2 fair sized onions sliced, and strain. This is an excellent salve for inflamed wounds. Apply twice or thrice daily, as needed.

❀

Salve, or Balsam, for Wounds, Cracks, or Internal Pains - Rosin, 2 1/2 lbs; spirits of turpentine, 1 qt; balsam of fir, 4 ozs; oil of hemlock, 2 ozs. Melt the rosin, and remove from the fire, then when a little cool, stir in the fir, turpentine, and last, the oil of hemlock, continuing to stir until cool enough to remain permanently mixed.

❀

Balm of Gilead Oil - Balm of Gilead buds any quantity; place them in a suitable dish for stewing, and pour upon them sufficient sweet oil to just cover them; stew thoroughly and press out all of the oil from the buds, and bottle for use. It will be found very valuable as a healing oil.

❀

Onion Salve - Slice a medium sized onion into 4 ounces of vaseline, stew together and strain. Apply two or three times a day to inflamed wounds.

❀

Salve for Cuts, Bruises and Corns - Take 1 pound each of rosin, beeswax and sheep's tallow and 1 1/4 pounds of raw linseed oil. Simmer down until of the proper consistency for a salve.

❀

Effectual Corn Salve - Simmer together a teaspoonful each of pine tar, brown sugar and saltpetre. After paring the corn, spread the salve on a piece of thin leather and bind on for two or three days. A piece of old kid glove will do nicely for the leather.

❀

Felon Salve - Shave some soap very fine, moisten with spirits of turpentine and apply to the felon. A fine salve for felons.

❀

Salve for Wounds, Burns and Old Sores - Take half a pound of beeswax, half a pound of salty butter, a quarter of a pound of turpentine and 6 ounces of balsam of fir. Simmer these together for half an hour and when cool the salve is ready for use.

Take one part (by weight) rosin, one part beeswax, and four parts good fresh sound lard. Mix and melt together over fire, so as to be sure not to burn the mixture. It makes an ointment that is superior for the flesh of either fresh or old sores, and especially good to remove old dry scabs. It softens the scab, and it comes off, leaving the skin soft.

❀

Camphor Ointment - 2/3 sliced camphor; 1/3 lard. Boil both together until the camphor is dissolved. It must be kept in a bottle with a glass stopper or something to prevent evaporation of camphor. It must be air tight or it will be good for nothing.

Sprains/Bruises

Wormwood boiled in vinegar and applied hot as can be borne on a sprain or bruise is an invaluable remedy. The affected member should afterwards be rolled in flannel to retain the heat.

❀

Take one part blue clay and two parts vinegar, and make into a paste, and bind on at night with a wet towel. One application is generally sufficient.

❀

Take cider vinegar, 1 pt; spirits of turpentine, 1/2 pt; beat well, 3 eggs, and mix all. Apply this to sprains or swellings by saturating (thoroughly wetting) cloths and lay on, or bind on when necessary.

❀

Mix equal parts of turpentine and coal oil and if for man add a little sweet oil to keep from blistering. This liniment is fine for all kinds of sprains, sores, swellings and frostbites in man or beast.

❀

The white of an egg, into which a piece of alum about the size of a hickory-nut has been stirred, stirring constantly until it forms a jelly or curd, is a capital remedy for sprains. It should be laid over the sprain upon a piece of lint, and be changed or re-wet in the whey as often as it becomes dry.

❀

When a beef was being dressed, the gall bladder was saved and the bile was drained into a bottle, then mixed with an equal part of turpentine. This makes a very healing liniment which can be used on many wounds and sprains.

Skin an eel in long strips and wrap it around as a bandage with the fat inside in. The eel fat soothes, and the skin being elastic will not bind too tightly.

Wounds/Bleeding

To stop bleeding, make a stiff paste of flour and vinegar and apply over the wound, binding on a piece of blotting paper.

❀

Brandy, or common whisky, 2 ozs; castile soap, 2 drams; carbonate of potash, 1 dram. Scrape the soap fine and dissolve it in the spirits; then add the potash; mix well and keep corked. Warm it and wet pledgets of lint in it and apply to the wound. It immediately congeals the blood and coagulates it some distance within the vessel. It may need repeating for deep wounds and when limbs are cut off.

❀

To stop the flow of blood from slight cuts a simple remedy is to bind the cut with cobwebs and brown sugar, pressed on like lint.

❀

Take the roots of bullrushes and bruise till it is like putty and apply to the effected parts in the case of blood poisoning.

❀

Dissolve 2 tablespoonfuls of epsom salts in 1 cup of boiling water. Soak a piece of bread into it, then place on the affected part as hot as can be borne. Change the bread every twenty minutes, until relief is obtained.

❀

A remedy for cuts and burns is glue and mucilage. This closes up a cut nicely, and one will experience no inconvenience thereafter. Cuts and burns are shorn of their terrors when the glue or mucilage is handy and ready for use.

❀

In all ordinary or slight cases of bleeding from the nose, cold water freely applied to the back of the neck, the face, and snuffed up the bleeding nostrils, will soon check it. However in severe cases, take a piece of very dry and hard salt beef, that which has been smoked is best, and grate it into a powder, and push this up the nostril, as far as possible, until it is filled, and let it remain. This never fails.

The leaves of the common geranium are an excellent remedy for cuts, or where the skin is rubbed off, and other wounds of that kind. One or two leaves, bruised and applied to the parts, and the wounds will be cicatrized (healed) in a short time.

❀

The bleeding of a wound on man or beast may be stopped by a mixture of wheat flour and common salt in equal parts, bound on with a cloth. If the bleeding be profuse, use a large quantity from one to three pints. It may be left for hours or even days. In this manner a horse was saved from bleeding from a wounded artery, which ceased in five minutes. It was left on for three days and soon healed.

❀

For bleeding, take linen or other rags, burn to charcoal and put it in the wound, and no more blood will come.

❀

In the case of wire cuts, take carbolic acid, 1 ounce; water, 1 pint; mix. Apply this to the cut three or four times a day until the cavity gets nearly full with new flesh, and then apply mutton tallow.

PAINTS AND COLORS. AYLMER, ONT.

ISAAC WILDERN,

VIENNA, ONT.

DEALER IN

DRUGS, MEDICINES AND CHEMICALS,

TOILET AND FANCY ARTICLES,

Sponges, Brushes, Perfumery, &c. Physicians' Prescriptions carefully compounded, and orders answered with care and dispatch. Farmers and Physicians from the country will find our stock of Medicines complete, warranted genuine, and of the best quality.

W. A. McCollom & Bro.,

TILSONBURG AND PORT BURWELL,

Advertisement, 1877

Miscellaneous

To Remove Black Specks or "Flesh worms" - Wash, and rub thoroughly with a towel and then apply the following twice a day—white brandy, 4 ozs; cologne, 2 ozs; liquor of potassa, 1 oz.

❀

Hiccoughs, to cure - Press the thumb of the right hand in the palm of the left, and hold the breath. If still had, try a pinch of salt, or swallow one teaspoonful of vinegar.

❀

Cramp Liniment - Heat 8 ounces of whisky or rum and pour upon half an ounce of cayenne. Dip cloths in this and apply to the affected parts and the pain of cramps will soon be relieved.

❀

Cure for Ague - Cut three lemons into thin slices and pound them with a mallet, then take enough coffee to make a quart, boil it down to a pint and pour it while quite hot over the lemons. Let it stand till cold, then strain through a cloth, and take the whole at one dose, immediately after the chill is over, and before the fever comes on.

❀

Cure for Drunkenness - Warranted a certain remedy. Confine the patient to his room, furnish him with his favourite liquor of discretion, diluted with 2/3 of water, as much wine, beer, coffee and tea as he desires, but containing 1/8 of spirit; all the food—the bread, meat and vegetables steeped in spirit and water. On the fifth day of this treatment he has an extreme disgust for spirit, being continually drunk. Keep up this treatment till he no longer desires to eat or drink, and the cure is certain.

❀

The passions and affections of the mind, viz. joy, fear, anger, etc., produce very sensible effects, and, when given too much way to, have a very bad effect on health, for they affect the stomach, hinder digestion, and chylification; whence arise many terrible disorders: wherefore it is best to keep them in bounds as much as possible, and to preserve an inward serenity, calmness, and tranquillity.

❀

To prevent bed sores, apply with a feather the white of an egg beaten with two teaspoonfuls spirits of wine.

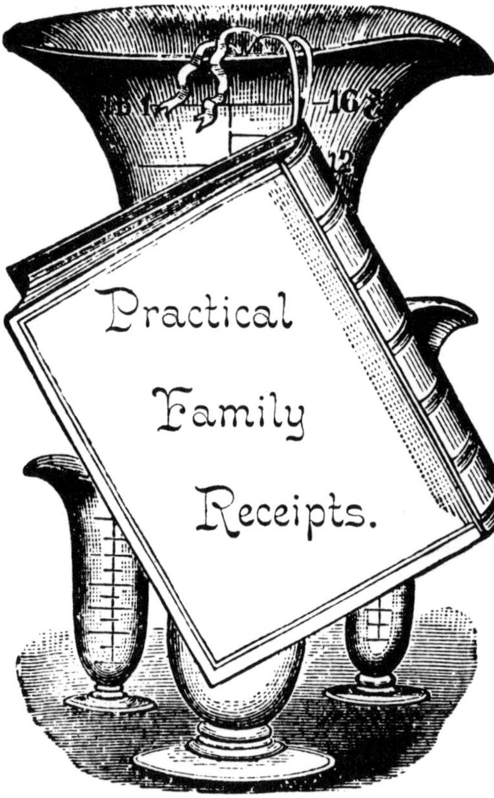

ALL KINDS OF FAMILY RECEIPTS AND REMEDIES.

An Infallible Cure for Lowness of Spirits - Take one ounce of spirits of resolution, an equal proportion of the oil of good conscience; infuse into these a tablespoonful of the salts of patience, and add thereto a few sprigs of others' woes, which grow extensively in the garden of life. Gather, also, a handful of the blossoms of hope; sweeten these with the balm of Providence, and, if possible, procure a few drops of genuine friendship, but be careful of counterfeits in the ingredient of self-interest, which grows spontaneously - the least admixture of it with the above would spoil the composition. Reduce the whole to an electuary by a proper proportion of content, flavour with the essence of good judgement, and regulate the quantity taken according to the virulence of the disease.

❀

To Distinguish Poison Bottles - When medicines have all to be kept in one place, and on one shelf. Round the neck of bottle labelled "Poison," tie a wee toy bell; the ringing of the bell will often prevent an accident.

In Case of Serious Illness - A bed of garden mould or sand laid on the hearth in front of a fire will prevent the noise of falling coal cinders from disturbing the patient.

❀

A bit of grated wild turnip, the size of a bean, and saturated with spirits of turpentine, for a felon.

❀

Carbuncles - Tomato poultice, thickened with powdered crackers has never been known to fail.

❀

Soot Coffee - Soot scraped from a chimney (that from stove pipes does not do), 1 tablespoon steeped in 1 pint of water, and settled with 1 egg beaten up in a little water, as for other coffee, with sugar and cream. Take three times daily with meals in place of other coffee. Used for cases of ague, jaundice, dyspepsia, typhoid fever, etc.

❀

Black heads - In a torpid condition of the skin there appears on the face, nose, and lower part of the forehead of many persons, what are called "black heads," "flesh worms," etc. - often in great numbers, and causing an exceedingly disagreeable appearance. When the skin is pressed with the finger-nails they come out in vermicular form, having a black point or head, which gives rise to the name grubs, or flesh worms, which they are, being real, living worms, which has been ascertained by microscopical examination. They can generally be permanently removed by pressing them out with the finger-nails, and then bathing the parts with mild salt water. The skin should receive gentle friction daily with a coarse towel.

❀

To fumigate a room with sulphur, use two pounds of rock sulphur with one pound of flowers of sulphur to every 1,000 cubic feet. Put the sulphur in a tin dish, set in a pan of wet ashes or a pan containing brick, to prevent any danger of fire. Put the rock sulphur at the bottom, the flowers of sulphur on top, and pour two tablespoonfuls of alcohol over them just before you apply the match. Leave the room instantly. Every door, window, crack and crevice in the room must be closed. It may discolour the paper. That depends on the colour. All the metal work must be removed.

Cooking For The Sick

Matters which might seem trivial to a well person are often of the greatest importance to one who is confined to his bed with sickness. A careless or wilful neglect of such details on the part of the nurse may cause what little appetite the patient has to disappear, while on the other hand, a careful observance of them may encourage a capricious desire for food into becoming a genuine and pleasurable appetite.

The Household Guide, 1899

Fresh water, a good sized cooking kettle and a reliable wood stove—these were the three basic necessities for the preparation of food for the sick as well as for the healthy.

A fourth necessity was that of ingenuity, particularly when preparing nourishing meals for those who had come down with debilitating ailments. The recipes for the unwell were varied, but the main ingredients were those which were common and readily available.

The combining of the ingredients at hand is where the caregiver was called upon to use her good sense and ingenuity to create nutritious and curative meals. Take, for example, the egg, which was one of the most common staples in the household. With an egg or two, and some milk and sugar brought to a boil, one could provide a soothing warm drink for a cough or cold. The same egg could be left to dissolve for several days in vinegar or lemon juice to provide a fortifying drink for the very weak.

Milk, chicken, beef and various herbs were equally common ingredients in recipes for the sick. Cooked slowly and strained, they could be made into a wide variety of teas and gruels which could be given to those too ill to take anything other than liquids. If left in more solid form (as in calf's foot jelly or oatmeal porridge), they were the main ingredients of meals served to the convalescent.

Perseverance and courage were two other ingredients which undoubtedly helped to sustain the patient as well as the caregiver. The following quotation from *Ye Old Miller's Household Book* (1899) sets a fitting context for the recipes which follow:

There is sickness everywhere, and as it falls to the lot of most women at some time in their lives to be nurse or cook for the sick, a few hints may be useful. Every woman with a tender, loving heart, no matter what her position, will try in such a case to tempt the appetite of the afflicted with her own delicate cooking and serving, the result being in many cases, returning health, and in any case having the satisfaction of knowing you have done what you could.

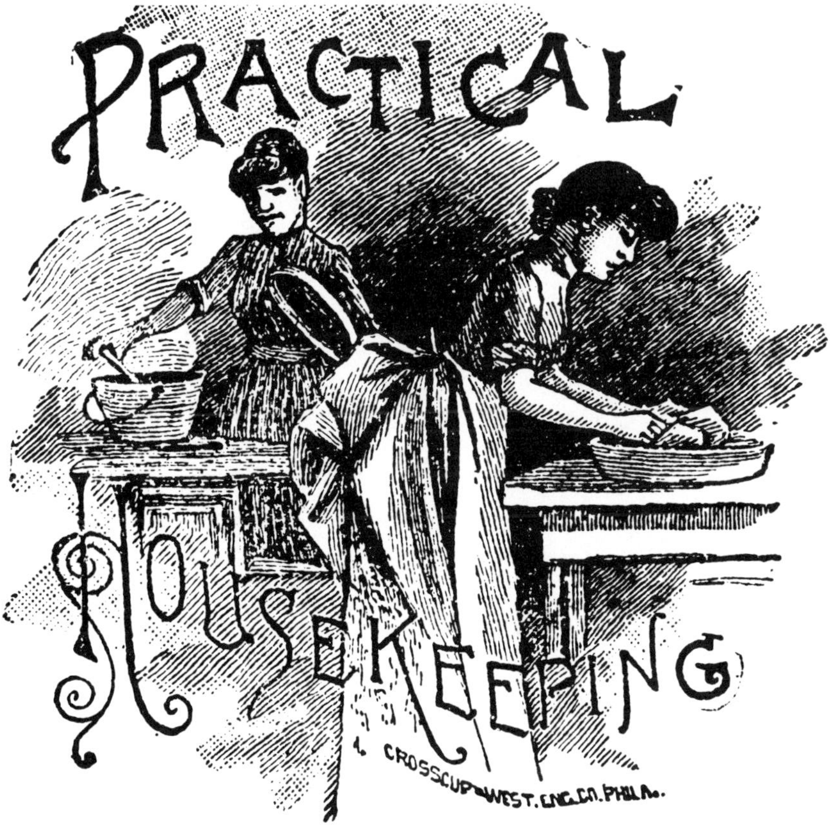

Practical Methods and Receipts for the Care of Kitchen Utensils.

In particular, the following rules were to be observed in preparing, cooking and serving food for the sick:

1. All the utensils employed should be scrupulously clean.

2. Never make a large quantity of one thing at a time.

3. Serve everything in as tempting and elegant a form as possible.

4. Put only a small quantity of an article on a dish at a time.
5. Keep milk and other delicacies on ice in warm weather.
6. Never leave food about a sick room.
7. Never offer beef tea or broth with the smallest particle of fat or grease on it, nor milk that is sour, nor meat or soup that is turned, nor an egg that is bad, nor vegetables that are underdone.

The Family Physician or Every Man His Own Doctor, 1909

Teas & Other Soothing Beverages

Beef Tea (Simplest way of making) - Cut the beef into very small pieces, and take away all the fat. Put it into a stone jar with a pint of water to each pound of beef; tie a double piece of brown paper over the top, and set the jar in a cool oven for several hours. Strain the beef tea off through a rather coarse strainer, and while it is hot take off every speck of fat with paper. If it is wanted stronger, put only half that amount of water. Should an oven be not obtainable, it will do equally well to place the jar in a large saucepan of boiling water; but it will not do to cook it in a metal saucepan without a jar, because an invalid's palate is very sensitive, and the tea is sure to acquire an unpleasant flavour. If in the place of lean beef some beef bones are used, the tea will become a jelly when cold; it will be less costly and less good. Any sort of flavouring may be added to it. A scrap of lemon-peel, a clove, a grate of nutmeg, a sprig of any sweet herb, or of parsley, put into the jar before cooking, will, any one of them, make a pleasant change, and a little ingenuity will soon increase the list. Such changes are grateful to a convalescent patient, and break the monotony of his life. However, a patient not decidedly convalescent needs nothing but beef and water, often not even salt. It is a lengthy process this, and if time is wanting to carry it out, twenty minutes is quite sufficient to set a cup of good beef tea on the table.

❀

Catnip Tea - It is considered, by old nurses, as the greatest panacea for infant ills.

❀

Mint Teas - From the dried or green leaves crushed, with a little sugar, are agreeable to the taste, and soothing to a nauseous stomach, and to an irritated condition of the bowels of children.

Flaxseed Lemonade - Pour one pint of boiling water over two tablespoons of whole flaxseed, when cool strain and add the juice of two lemons, and two tablespoons honey. Used for coughs, colds and suppressed urine.

❀

Apple Water - Cut two large apples in slices, and pour a quart of boiling water on them; or on roasted apples; strain in two or three hours, and sweeten slightly.

❀

Barley Water for the Sick or Nursing Mothers - Thoroughly wash two ounces of barley, to remove any musty or bad flavour; put in a clean pot on the fire, with two quarts of cold water, and boil it until it is reduced to one quart; then strain it, and let it cool; add a little sugar. A slice of lemon, or an apple cut in slices, may be added if liked. The barley can be used for soup, or made into a pudding.

❀

Toast and Water - Toast slowly a thin piece of bread till extremely brown and hard, but not the least black; then plunge it into a jug of cold water, and cover it over an hour before used. This is of particular use in weak bowels. It should be of a fine brown colour before drinking it.

❀

Buttermilk - For some forms of dyspepsia, in fevers, and in cases of diabetes buttermilk is an excellent food. May be sealed like fruit in glass jars and kept some time.

❀

Egg with Tea, Coffee, Cocoa or Milk - Break the egg into a teacup, beat with a fork till well mixed. Pour in the tea, coffee, cocoa, or milk, gradually stirring all the time. This is very nourishing and good in cases of exhaustion from over-work or mental strain.

❀

Eggs and Sherry - Beat up, with a fork, an egg till it froths, add a lump of sugar and two tablespoonfuls of water. Mix well. Then pour in a wineglassful of sherry, and serve before it gets flat. Half the quantity of brandy may be used instead of sherry.

This is a valuable preparation in cases of great prostration, when stimulants and concentrated nutriment are required.

A Nice Drink for a Cough - Ingredients: A fresh laid egg, 1/4 pint of new milk warmed, a large spoonful of capillaire, the same of rose-water, a little grated nutmeg.

Beat the egg and mix with remaining ingredients. Do not warm it after the egg has been put in.

❀

For Very Weak Invalids - Six fresh eggs, shells unbroken, cover with the juice of twelve lemons. Let digest for several days, then remove all pieces of skin or undissolved shell, after which pour over the mass one pint of rum and beat thoroughly; melt in a little water one pound of rock candy, and add after cooling, then bottle, and use a few spoonfuls. It will be found excellent and very nourishing.

❀

A Great Restorative - Bake two calf's-feet in two pints of water and the same quantity of new milk, in a jar, close-covered, three hours and a half. When cold, remove the fat.

❀

Sippets, when the stomach will not receive meat - On an extremely hot plate put two or three sippets of bread, and pour over them some gravy from beef, mutton, or veal, with which no butter has been mixed. Sprinkle a little salt over.

Jellies

Beef Jelly For Invalids - Three small onions, three small or one and one-half large carrots, a few whole cloves and black pepper, one small teaspoon of sugar, one slice of ham, two calf's feet, one and one-half pounds of beef. Put in the onions and other ingredients in succession. Place the ham on top, then the calf's feet, and lastly the beef; no water; put on the side of the range, and let it stand until reduced to a soft mass, then add a quart of water and let it boil one hour; strain and let stand until cold, then take off the fat. Use by dissolving a little in hot water.

❀

Pork Jelly (Dr. Ratcliffe's Restorative) - Ingredients: A leg of well-fed pork, 3 gals. of water, 1/2 oz. of mace, the same of nutmeg, salt to taste.

Take the pork just as cut up, beat it, and break the bone. Set it over a gentle fire with the water and simmer until it is reduced to one gallon. Let the mace and nutmeg stew with it. Strain through a fine sieve. When cold take off the fat. Give a large cupful the first and last thing and at noon, putting salt to taste.

❀

Tapioca Jelly - Ingredients: Some of the largest kind of tapioca, some lemon juice, wine, and sugar.

Pour cold water on to wash it two or three times, then soak it in fresh water five or six hours, and simmer it in the same until quite clear; then add the lemon juice, wine, and sugar. The peel should have been boiled in it. It thickens very much.

Gruels & Other Nourishing Dishes

Effervescing Gruel - Ingredients: Half a breakfast cup of thin water gruel, 1 tablespoonful of sifted white sugar, a saltspoonful of carbonate of soda, juice of a lemon.

Mix the soda and sugar well together and then put into the gruel, stirring thoroughly; have ready the lemon juice strained, throw it in and drink immediately while it is effervescing and as hot as possible.

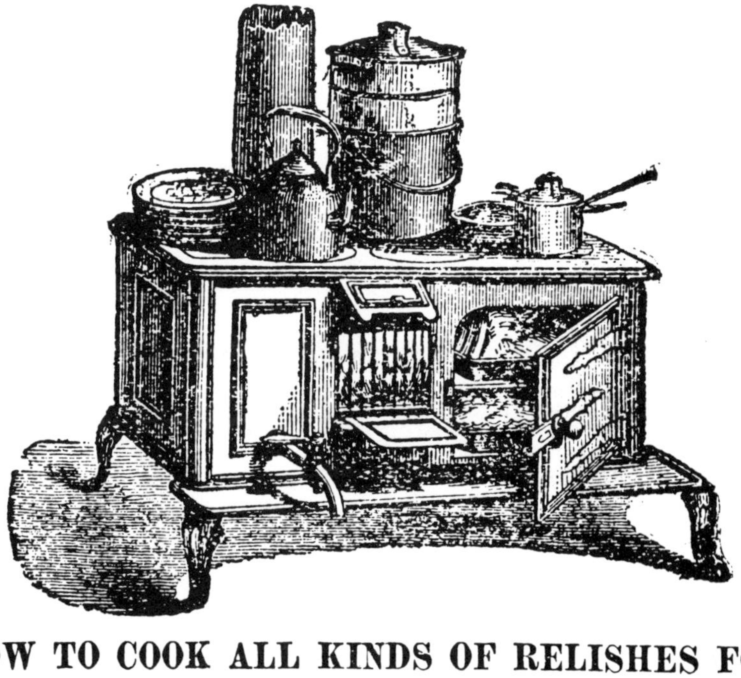

HOW TO COOK ALL KINDS OF RELISHES FOR THE SICK.

Egg Gruel - Boil eggs from one to three hours until hard enough to grate; then boil new milk and thicken with the egg, and add a little salt. Excellent in cases of nausea.

❀

Oatmeal Porridge or Gruel - Mix 2 tablespoons of the finely ground oatmeal with a little cold water, then stir it into 1 pt. of boiling water and let it boil 15 or 20 minutes. Add a little salt and sugar to taste; if desired a small quantity of wine and nutmeg may also be added.

❀

Pap, or Boiled Flour - Tie 1 cup of flour closely in a cloth, and boil 5 hours; when cool grate off a tablespoonful of it, and mix smoothly in a little cold milk; then stir this mixture into 1 pt. of boiling milk, and boil a few minutes, and sweeten with loaf sugar, and add a little nutmeg, if desired. Very valuable in diarrhoea of children or adults.

❀

Cracked or Rolled Wheat - Cracked wheat should be stirred into boiling water and cooked in a double kettle for 3 hours. Salt and serve either hot or cold in moulds with fruit sauce or cream and sugar. Rolled wheat may be cooked the same way, only it does not require to cook so long. Do not soak in cold water, but stir into boiling water, as all the grains should be. Wheat is excellent for constipation or biliousness.

❀

Custard - One egg, gill of milk, teaspoonful sugar. Have a pan on the fire with boiling water, put the milk in a jug (or jelly can), and set it in the water; beat up the egg very light, and add it to the milk with the sugar, and stir till it sets; remove it from the boiling water, and serve (or it can be browned before the fire).

❀

Scotch Broth - Ingredients: The liquor in which a leg of mutton, piece of beef, or old fowl has been boiled, barley, vegetables chopped small, a cup of rough oatmeal mixed in cold water, salt and pepper to taste.

Add to the liquor some barley and vegetables, chopped small, in sufficient quantity to make the broth quite thick. The necessary vegetables are carrots, turnips, onions, and cabbage, but any others may be added; old (not parched) peas and celery are good additions. When the vegetables are boiled tender, add the oatmeal to the broth, salt and pepper to taste. This very plain preparation is genuine Scotch broth as served in Scotland; with any colouring or herbs, etc., added, it is not real Scotch broth. It is extremely palatable and wholesome in its plain form.

The matter of diet requires great attention. Sick people have very frequently very delicate and very capricious appetites. They take a fancy to a thing, and, if they could have it quickly, would greatly relish it, but if they have to wait an hour or two, the inclination evaporates, and when it is ready, the desire for it is gone. Again; many people have not judgement, and will present a sick person with a mess, "fit," according to the old expression, "for a plough-boy." The very sight of such a quantity destroys the appetite, while a small portion of the same would have been taken and enjoyed.

Smith's Family Physician, 1869.

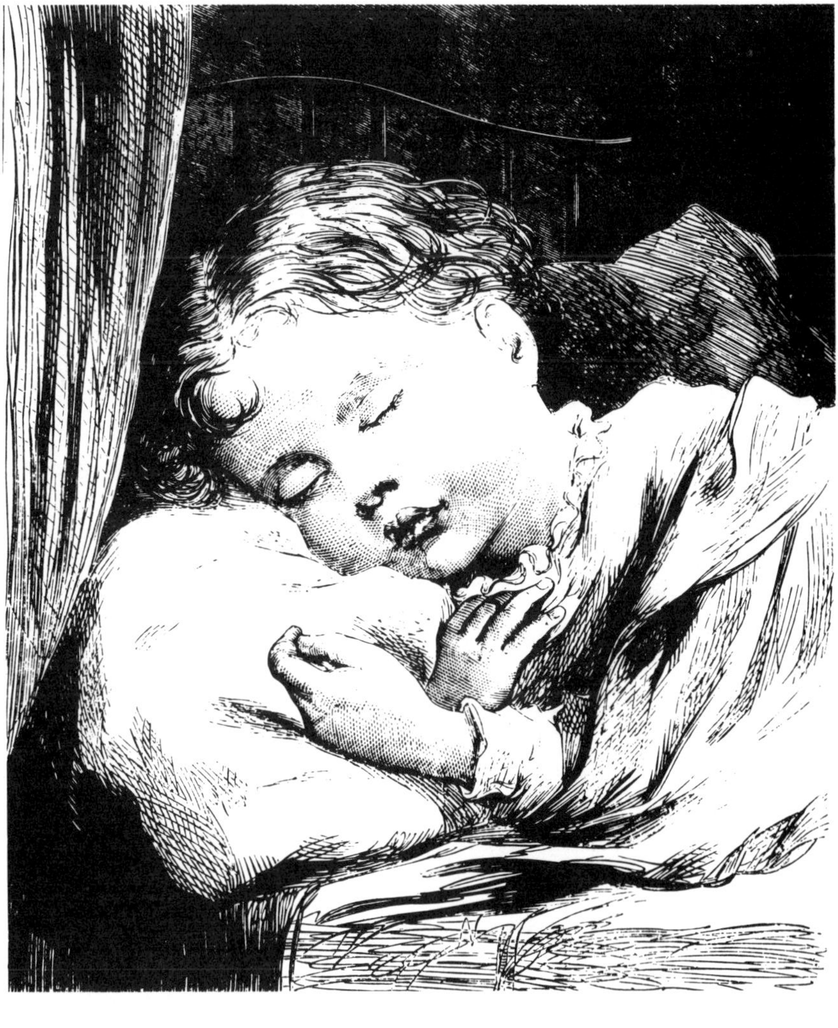

Dr. Taylor of Innerkip

In 1885 a book was published in Woodstock, Ontario, entitled *The Medical Recipes of the late Doctor Taylor of Innerkip* (published, according to instructions left by him, by George Hotson and James Miller).

Who was Dr. Taylor of Innerkip? Perhaps this is only an interesting and somewhat obtuse enquiry—yet it leads to another view of minority medicine during this period.

The *County of Oxford Directory for 1874* identified Innerkip as a post village in the Township of East Zorra, situated on the western bank of the Thames River, eight miles from the county town of Woodstock. The population of the village was 200, and contained two stores, two hotels, a blacksmith and a wagon shop, a school with an average attendance of 80 pupils and two churches (Presbyterian and Church of England). A Baptist congregation was situated on the 16th Concession, a short distance from the village. Manufacturing in the village consisted of an oatmeal mill (erected in 1860), employing both steam and water power, a flour and grist mill (built in 1864) with a capacity of 50 barrels per day, and several lime kilns which turned out 100 bushels every 12 hours.

Residents of Innerkip included several blacksmiths, butchers, teachers, labourers, carpenters/coopers, and a wagon maker as well as Mrs. Sarah Begg (post mistress and general store), the Rev. Samuel H. Freshneyer (pastor, Baptist church), and John Taylor (root and herb doctor).

The 1867 *Gazetteer* for Oxford and Norfolk Counties listed Dr. Taylor, "coloured" in Innerkip. The 1871 census of the Dominion of Canada provides a few more details. John Taylor, age 67, is listed as a root doctor, birth place—the West Indies, religion—regular Baptist. He was enumerated with this wife, Nancy (age 62), born in the West Indies, and a daughter, Elizabeth (age 21), single.

The Woodstock Sentinel Review of April 4, 1884 noted under deaths:

> Taylor—on the 28th of March, at Innerkip, Dr. John Taylor, root and herb doctor, at the age of 81 years.

What else do we know about John Taylor? The publisher's preface to the book of 1885 notes that:

> For the last twenty-three years Taylor has been looked upon as a necessity by scores of invalids. His wonderful cures of chronic and dangerous diseases, after the cases had been given up by the profession, are so well known that a repetition of the cases is needless.
>
> Some of his cures he learned from his father, a pure African doctor; others he picked up from various sources. Thompson and Culpeper were his standard authorities. Up to within a year of his death he experimented on everything new that he met with, generally to throw it away as worthless. But whenever he met with anything good he entered it on his books. It cannot be said that there is anything new in his cures. Their chief value consists in their simplicity, and the fact that they are the doctor's gems of seventy years' practice.

John Taylor was clearly an adherent to the Thompsonian (botanic) School as he notes in the author's preface:

> I am one of the few who believe that in every country there are herbs to cure every disease natural to that country, if we only knew them. Few people are aware of the value of some of the simple herbs growing around their doors. If they did they would put greater value upon them. You can scarcely walk across your back yard without tramping over some of the most valuable remedies for kidney and other diseases.

In the preface, he discusses at some length his criticism of and antipathy towards the established medical community, and their treatments:

> Why do we boast that this is the land of freedom if we dare not as free and independent people think and act for ourselves? When our legislators throw the shield of law around a person of monopoly, when that monopoly is moreover inimical to the wishes of the people and the best interests of the community, do our legislators act wisely and disinterestedly to the community at large?
>
> Why does the apothecary color and disguise his drugs? Why does a physician prescribe in bad Latin? These artifices are resorted to in order to deceive the public. Now these poor patients would tremble if they knew the nature of the compounds administered. Deadly poisons are administered for almost every disease.

John Taylor describes a recent incident when he was charged before a magistrate with violating the Medical Act: "Observe, I was not charged with having injured any person." Apparently, an individual was being treated by "certain of the protected medical profession" who concluded that the only way to save the patient's life was to amputate his leg. As a last resort, the man sent for Taylor, who saved both his life and limb, "and to the astonishment, and I doubt not chagrin, of these protected monopolists that individual is alive and well today."

John Taylor, as best as one can describe him, was certainly an interesting if not a unique individual. Not in the sense of being a member of the botanic school of healing, but as a black West Indian living and having an important role in a small rural community in southwestern Ontario long before the end of the 19th century. His story illustrates not only the many and varied ways in which families and communities dealt with self-help medicine, but also the negative opinions about the main stream medical profession of the day.

In his book, Taylor describes in detail a range of readily available herbs with particulars of their doses and uses. What follows is a selection of some of his "medical recipes."

> These remedies for the cure of the sick and afflicted have been entrusted to me by a kind and beneficent Providence, who will hold me accountable for the manner in which I have used them. And although I have been very successful in the healing art, remember that I have only been an instrument in the hands of an over-ruling Providence.
>
> Convinced as I am of the truth of these remarks, I know that I would not be fulfilling the trust reposed in me by a good and kind Providence if I did not publish to the world those great remedies and cures which have been entrusted to me and for which I will be held accountable.

How To Make Number Six

This medicine is to remove pain and prevent mortification, to be taken or applied externally, or to be put into the injections. One or two teaspoonfuls of this medicine may be given alone or the same quantity may be put into other medicines. It may also be used to bathe with in all cases of external swellings or pains. It is an excellent remedy for rheumatism by taking a dose and also bathing the parts affected with it. For the headache by taking a swallow and bathing the head and snuffing a little up the nose.

It is good for bruises, sprains, swelled joints and cold sores, it will allay the inflammation, bring down swelling, ease pain and produce a tendency to heal, in fact there is hardly a complaint in which this useful medicine cannot be used to advantage. It is the best preservative against mortification of anything I have ever found.

Take one gallon of fourth proof brandy or high wines, one pound of gum myrrh pounded fine and one ounce of Cayenne pepper, put them into a stone jug, boil it twenty minutes in a kettle of water leaving the jug uncorked; when settled bottle for use. For external application add a little turpentine and a little gum camphor. It may be prepared without boiling by letting it stand in the jug for five or six days, shaking it well every day. It will then be fit for use.

Colic

Blue or White Belmonie Root, Swamp Milkweed Root, equal parts, steeped in hot water; sweeten to taste. Take dry black cherries pounded to a powder, tincture in brandy, half a pound of powder to a quart of brandy. Dose, from one teaspoonful to one tablespoonful, according to strength of patient; add the tincture in proportion of one quarter to three quarters of the decoction. This is to regulate the stomach and digestive organs.

Bleeding At Nose

Puff Ball, snuff the dust. Also take a woman's apron, steep in cold water and apply it to the privates. This is a speedy and effectual remedy.

Putrid Sore Throat

One pound of the root of Golden Rod, bruised, put into one gallon soft water, boil down one half, strain, then boil down to one quart; keep the vessel covered while boiling; when taken off the fire, add half ounce Burnt Alum, half ounce Borax, quarter teaspoonful of Cayenne pepper, one tablespoonful Number Six. When cool bottle for use. Gargle the throat with this mixture and spit it out; use it freely as it will not hurt anyone.

Dyspepsia

Horseradish cut fine, tincture in Whisky, add a little Cayenne pepper. Dose, a tablespoonful three times a day.

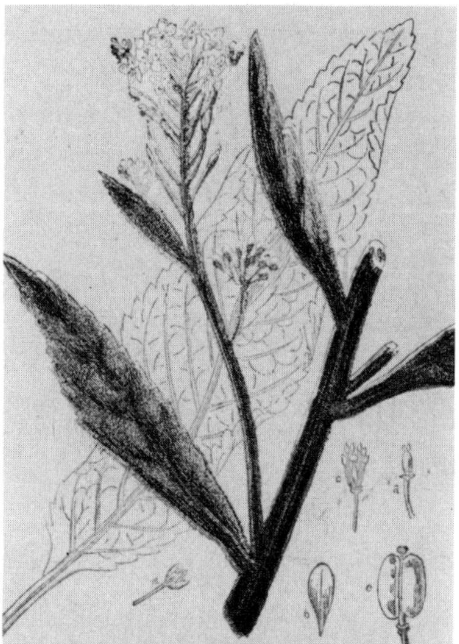

Horse-radish.

Cancer

Take a large sugar kettle, fill it with pine boughs, boil in soft water until the boughs become yellow, than take out the boughs and fill again and boil as before, then strain it off, boil the juice down to the consistency of tar, add one pound hog's lard, one pound mutton tallow, one pound beef tallow, one pound resin, one pound of turpentine from pine tree, half ounce saltpetre, one ounce burnt alum, half ounce burnt copperas, one pound beeswax. Simmer over a slow fire, stirring all the time, twelve hours; before taking off add one tablespoonful of sulphur. Be careful not to burn. Strain while hot through a fine wire sieve. When you use it, spread it on a piece of leather a little larger than the cancer.

Consumption

Take 2 ounces of turpentine from pine tree, half a pound of sugar, put them into a quart of gin, bottle up. Mix them well and shake well before using. Dose, one tablespoonful four times a day before eating and before going to bed.

Canker

1. Bayberry root bark, white pond lily root and the inner bark of hemlock, equal parts of each, pounded and well mixed together. Steep one ounce of the powder in a pint of boiling water and give for a dose a common wineglassful sweetened to taste.

2. Red raspberry leaves, white pond lily roots, witch hazel leaves or bark, golden root, white mullen, wild flax, hemlock bark, red oak bark, white oak bark, Solomon's Seal, equal parts. Boil well, then strain and simmer down strong. Sweeten to taste. Dose, tablespoonful three or four times a day.

Dropsy

1. Pond lily, one pound; milk weed root, one pound; chamomile flowers, half ounce. Boil them in one gallon of water; strain and boil down to one quart. When cold add a half pint of gin or brandy. Dose, tablespoonful every four hours.

2. Take a gallon of the best apple vinegar; put it into a vessel; fill it up with old, rusty iron; let it stand twelve hours. Dose, half a teacupful every four hours.

3. Burn one pound of grape vines to ashes. Put the ashes into half a gallon of sweet wine. Dose, a half teacupful every four hours.

Cough Syrup

1. One pound poplar bark, one pound of bayberry; boil them in two gallons of water; strain and add half a teaspoonful of lobelia and a teaspoonful of Number Six. Dose, commence with a tablespoonful twice a day and increase to half a wineglassful.

2. Indian turnip, boneset, lobelia leaves, elecampane, each one ounce, hoarhound, skunk cabbage, each two ounces, blood root, half ounce. Pound them all up and mix thoroughly. Dose, from one teaspoonful to half a wineglassful twice a day.

3. Pine boughs and pine burrs; boil down strong; then strain; add one pound of sugar to every two quarts of juice; simmer down into a syrup; stir while boiling. Dose, half a teaspoonful for a child; for an adult, one tablespoonful night and morning.

Rheumatism

1. Quarter pound of white cohosh root, quarter pound queen of the meadow, quarter teaspoonful of Cayenne pepper. Put all into a quart of best whiskey. Dose, wineglassful three times a day. Also rub the part affected with Number Six.

2. Saltpetre, half ounce; spirits of turpentine, one ounce; beef gall, three ounces; high wine, one ounce. Mix all well together and rub the place well. Rub also with high wines and Cayenne pepper.

Nerve Ointment

Take bark of the root of bitter sweet, two parts; of wormwood and chamomile each one part. If dry moisten with hot water; then put into horse, porpoise, or any other kind of soft animal oil and simmer them over a slow fire for twelve hours; then strain it off and add one ounce of spirits of turpentine to each pound of ointment. To be used for a bruise, sprain, callous swelling, or for corns.

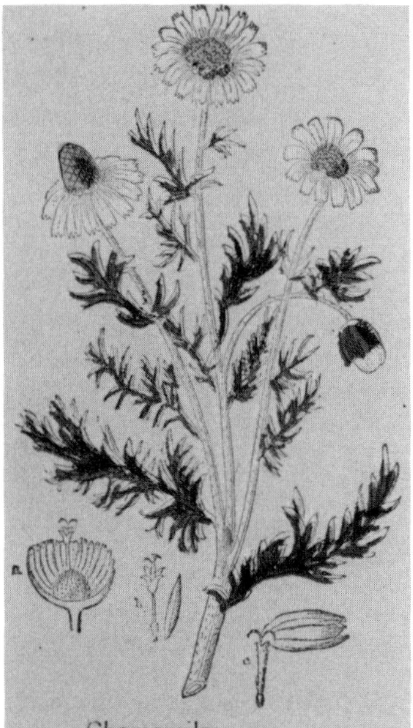
Chamomile.

Ointment For The Eyes

Celandine (or touch-me-not) roots and tops, bruise them down, then squeeze out all the juice and mix hog's grease with it and stew them into an ointment and anoint the eyes with it.

Poultice

Make a strong tea of raspberry leaves. Take a cracker pounded fine and slippery elm bark pulverized with ginger and make a poultice of the same. This is good for sores, felons, and for bad burns, scalds and parts frozen. Apply this poultice and renew it at least as often as every twelve or twenty-four hours and wash with soap suds at every renewal, wetting in the interim with cold water or a tea of raspberry leaves.

Women in Travail

One handful of red raspberry leaves, half a handful of blue Cohosh steeped as tea; add a little sweet milk, a little sugar and a little cayenne pepper. This tea is good both before and after birth. Take a teaspoonful of umbel or lady's slipper, draw by itself like tea. Put a teaspoonful into a half teacupful of the syrup and add a few drops of Number Six. These will allay the after pains, cause cheerfulness and give strength. Half a teacupful of the syrup to be taken at two doses.

Piles

1. Strong decoction of yarrow herb tea; take out the herbs and boil strong. Dose, wineglass three times a day.
2. Take a rind of old bacon, the older the better, cut into small pieces, put live coals into a pot; put the bacon rind on coals, smother them so that they will not blaze; then take a stool with a hole in the bottom, set the vessel under and wrap a cloth round the stool so that the smoke cannot escape and let the patient sit on the stool. Continue until relieved. I have never known this to fail.
3. Take about eight or nine inches of the end of the large gut of a pig; let fat and everything remain on and in it, just in its natural state; put it into a pan and fry it out until perfectly brown, chop it up while frying, strain it off, squeeze all the fat out of it, bottle up and ready for use. Apply to the part with the finger.
4. Take the root of the skunk cabbage, the male root. This root grows like a carrot in wet land. Wash it clean, split it open, scrape out the inside, put it into a cloth, squeeze the juice out, mix the juice with hog's lard, then stew it well, then bottle for use. This ointment must be applied with the finger both inside and outside.

Liniment

Two ounces of the best gum myrrh well pulverized, oil of hemlock one ounce, cayenne pepper, gum camphor and oil organum, of each half an ounce, balsam of fir, half ounce. Add a little spirit of turpentine and about as much saltpetre as will lie on a five cent piece. Mix all in a pint of alcohol, let stand five or six days before using, shaking well each day. This liniment is good for relieving pain in all parts of the body. To be applied to the parts affected with a feather.

Diabetes

The hind claws of a hog; grind them to a powder; then take one teaspoonful of the powder in one tablespoonful of vinegar to a dose, three times a day.

The *Canada Farmer*

The mid to the late 19th century saw the emergence, if not the initial flourishing, of the newspaper age in Canada. The increasing population and growing prosperity of the more settled parts of the country provided an expanded and more varied readership. While the majority of the papers were small local and urban weeklies, others tended to be more focused on rural and agricultural issues.

The *Canada Farmer* was a fortnightly paper with the subtitle, a *Journal of Agriculture, Horticulture and Rural Affairs*. It was owned and published by George Brown (who had founded *The Globe* in 1844) from 26 and 28 King Street East, Toronto, Canada West. It first appeared in 1864, coincidentally the same year that George Brown was to play a central role at the Charlottetown and Quebec Conferences leading to Confederation in 1867. The paper noted that "no exertion or expenditure will be spared to render the new Journal a worthy representative and advocate of the Agricultural interests of Canada" and that it was "the best and cheapest paper for the Canadian farmer." Indeed, its annual subscription was $1.00.

As was typical of the period, the paper republished material from a range of sources, e.g., other newspapers and books as well as from a wide variety of correspondents. Its main focus was on the rural reader and contained information on agricultural items—commodity prices, machinery, agricultural shows, crop production, and animal husbandry. The paper's first issue of January 15, 1864, under the section entitled "The Household," commented as follows:

> The maxim, "if a man would succeed well in his livelihood, he must ask his wife", is more applicable, perhaps, to the farmer's calling than to any other. No matter how well things may be carried on out of doors, unless there be thrifty and judicious management within doors, all will go wrong. The exercise of skill, prudence and good judgement on the part of the farmer's wife, is called for in a great variety of ways.

The *Canada Farmer* regularly contained a wide mixture of information and advice to its readers on domestic or household items—cooking, cleaning, preserving, home remedies, good health, and general social advice. The following is a rather varied selection from some of this material.

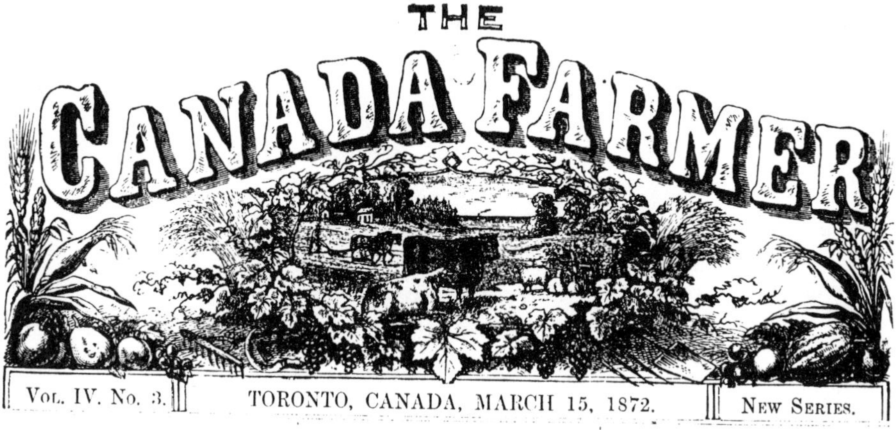

Children's Feet - Life long discomfort, disease, and death often come to children through the inattention, or carelessness of the parents. A child should never be allowed to go to sleep with cold feet; the thing to be last attended to, in putting a child to bed, should be to see that the feet are dry and warm; neglect of this has often resulted in a dangerous attack of croup, diphtheria, or fatal sore throat. Tight shoes inevitably arrest the circulation of the blood and nervous influences through the feet, and directly tend to cause cold feet; and health with habitually cold feet is an impossibility.

April 1, 1864

❀

Frosted Feet - Raw cotton and castor oil are said to be an infallible remedy for frozen limbs, and to have effected a cure when amputation was thought to be necessary to save life.

April 1, 1864

❀

A Novel Cure - It is said a poultice of onions, tobacco and salt, mixed in equal parts, bound tightly upon the part afflicted, is effectual in curing the bite of a rattlesnake or mad dog. It is worth remembering, as it may do good, and cannot do harm.

April 1, 1864

Useful Hints - Never enter a sick room in a state of perspiration, as the moment you become cool your pores absorb. Do not approach contagious diseases with an empty stomach; nor sit between the sick and the fire, because the heat attracts the thin vapour.

April 1, 1864

❀

Treatment Of Hiccups - This may often be removed by holding the breath, by swallowing a piece of bread, by sudden fright, or a draught of weak liquid. When it arises from heat and acidity in the stomachs of children, a little rhubarb and chalk will remove it. Should it proceed from irritability of nerves, take a few drops of sal volatile, with a teaspoonful of paregoric elixir. If it still continues, rub on soap liniment mixed with tincture of opium, or a plaster may be put on the pit of the stomach, or sipping a glass of cold water with a little carbonate of soda dissolved in it.

April 15, 1864

❀

Woollen Clothing - The healthful clothing for our climate, the year round, is that made of wool. If worn next to the skin by all classes, in summer as well as in winter, an incalculable amount of coughs, colds, diarrhoeas, dysenteries, and fever would be prevented by the ability of a woollen garment to keep the natural heat about the body more perfectly, instead of conveying it away as fast as generated, as linen and flaxen garments do; as also cotton and silk, although these are less cooling than Irish linen, as any one can prove by noticing the different degrees of coldness on the application of a surface six inches square of cotton flannel and linen to the skin, the moment the clothing is removed. The explanation is, that wool is a bad conductor of heat, and linen is good conductor.

In the night-sweats of consumption or of any debilitated condition of the system, a woollen flannel nightdress is immeasurably more comfortable than cotton or linen, because it prevents that sepulchral dampness and chilliness of feeling, which is otherwise inevitable.

The British government made it imperative that every sailor in the navy shall wear woollen flannel shirts in the hottest climate.

May 2, 1864

Diseases of the Kidney, Liver, Etc. - As a medicinal remedy in diseases of the kidneys, liver, stomach, etc., the dandelion is admitted to be excellent and being found on almost every cleared plot of land, it is within the reach of all. As a beverage it is equal in flavour to the best coffee, and few who use it for a month will be willing to give it up; it requires less sugar and half the quantity of the coffee. It is made by just washing the roots thoroughly, cut fine, dry near the stove for a while, then finish in the oven, add a little butter, and roast till brown, then grind in a coffee-mill. It is but little trouble, and you are sure the article is genuine. When bought from the shop it is likely to be four-fifths pea or rye meal.

May 2, 1864

❀

How To Cook a Husband - Many good husbands are spoiled in the cooking; some women go about as if they were bladders, and blow them up; others keep them constantly in hot water, while others freeze them by conjugal coolness; some smother them in hatred, contention and variance, and some keep them in pickle all their lives. These women always serve them up with tongue sauce. Now it cannot be supposed that husbands will be tender and good if managed in this way; but on the contrary, very delicious if managed as follows: Get a jar, called the jar of faithfulness (which all good wives keep on hand), place your husband in it, and set him near the fire of conjugal love. Let the fire be pretty hot, but especially let it be clear, and above all let the fire be constant. Cover him with affection, kindness and subjection, garnish with modest becoming familiarity, and spiced with pleasantry, and if you add kisses and other confectionaries, let them be accompanied with a sufficient portion of secrecy, mixed with prudence, and moderation. We would advise all good wives to try this recipe, and realize what an admirable dish a husband makes when properly cooked.

May 16, 1864

❀

How To Get Rid of Ants - Take sage and strew small quantities where they frequent. We have never yet failed of getting rid of them, not for a day or two only, but for the entire summer. Try it, you that are plagued with them, and we warrant you success. We hear much about camphor, but that, with us, never yet proved successful.

May 16, 1864

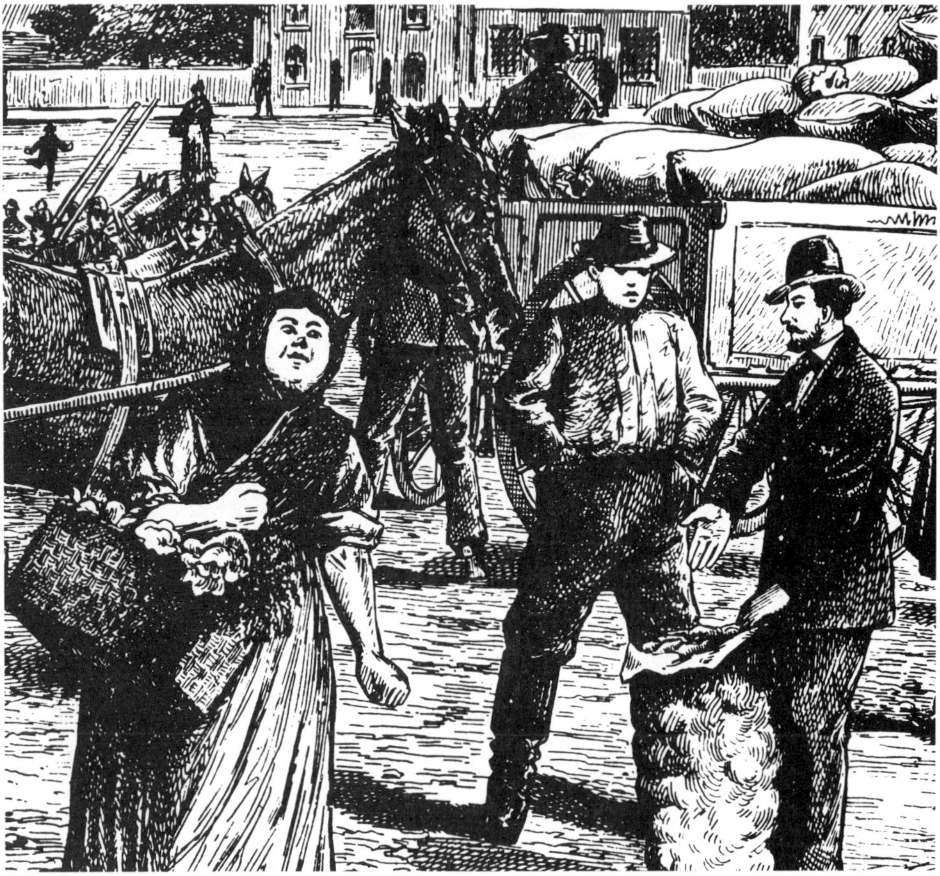

To Stop Bleeding of the Nose - Extraordinary as it may appear, a piece of brown paper, folded and placed between the upper lip and gum, it is said, will stop bleeding of the nose.

May 16, 1864

❀

Burns or Scalds - Maple molasses spread on a fine greasy cloth, and renewed when dry, cured a little child when badly scalded on the arm and breast. A piece of maple sugar boiled in sufficient water will do miracles. Mothers, try it and you will be thankful.

May 16, 1864

❀

Poison - If a person swallows poison deliberately or by chance, instead of breaking out into multitudinous and incoherent exclamations, despatch someone for the doctor. Meantime, run to the kitchen, get half a glass of water in anything that is handy, put into it a teaspoonful of salt, and as much ground mustard; stir it an instant, catch a firm hold of the person's nose; the mouth will soon fly open—then down with the mixture, and in a second or two up will come the poison.

June 15, 1864

❀

Cancer - Take a quantity of red oak bark, burnt to ashes; to this add water; boil to the consistency of molasses; apply to the part affected; leave on for an hour; afterwards cover the plaster with tar; remove in a few days, and if protuberances appear in the wound, apply the plaster and tar alternately until they all disappear, after which apply any healing salve.

June 15, 1864

❀

Blistered Hands and Feet - The speediest remedy is to light a tallow candle and let the melted tallow drop in cold water; then mix the tallow with strong spirits, and rub it thoroughly into the palms or soles; this is both a preventive and curative.

June 15, 1864

❀

A New Remedy For Tapeworm - Mash up into a cake with two ounces of honey, three ounces of pumpkin seed. This cake is to be eaten an hour before the usual time for breakfast, of which very little should be taken; if none be taken, all the better. An hour after the cake has been eaten, take two ounces more of honey, and an hour after that two ounces more. This should be tried for two days if necessary, and then, after an interval of a week, try again.

December 1, 1864

❀

Bed-bugs - They can be kept away by washing the crevices with strong salt water, put on with a brush.

January 2, 1865

❀

Diabetes - The cure of this disease is now effected in a very simple manner. It is this: Taking of fresh bran or yeast three or four times a day, at the same time meeting the waste produced by the disease on the system by the free use of Dublin porter, and all the solid nourishing food the patient can take.

January 16, 1865

Toothache - Place a little scraped horseradish in the mouth, or the tooth, and just around the gum. It relieves rheumatic pains in the gums and face also. The mouth may afterwards be rinsed with a little camphorated water, lukewarm.

February 1, 1865

❀

Efficacy Of Onions - A writer says: We are often troubled with severe coughs the results of colds of long standing, which may turn to consumption or premature death. Hard coughs cause sleepless nights by constant irritation in the throat, and a strong effort to throw off offensive matter from the lungs. The remedy I propose has been tried by me and I often recommend it to others with good results, which is simply to take into the stomach before retiring for the night, a piece of raw onion, after chewing. This esculent, in an uncooked state, is very healing, and tends to collect the water from the lungs and throat, causing immediate relief to the patient. Sliced onion, in a raw state, will collect poison from the air, and also from the human system when taken internally or externally applied to the arm pits.

February 1, 1865

❀

Cure For Frost Bites, Burns and Scalds - "D.B." sends the following: "Steep a piece of lime for six hours, and then for every two spoonsful of water, add one of linseed oil; stir until it becomes an ointment of the substance of cream, and then apply to the place affected. This is well worthy of a trial."

March 1, 1865

❀

Cleanliness and Health - Those to whom sanitary reform must be preached, are school-children. They should be taught, if we are dirty, we shall become diseased; if we sin, we shall suffer, as certainly as twice two are four, and twice four are eight. It is in the minds of little children that we should sow this seed.

March 15, 1865

❀

Cure For Bee Stings - From the *Prairie Farmer* we learn, on the authority of Dr. Bush, Chester Co., Pa., that one drop of strong spirits of hartshorn will in an instant remove the pain caused by the sting of a bee, wasp, or hornet. It should be at hand in every family where there are children. Smiles of gratitude, shining through the tears of distress, will often repay the thoughtful mind that provides and the quick hand that applies the remedy. He recommends the same article also for the removing of grease spots.

August 1, 1865

❀

How To Get Rid Of Mosquitoes - The *Maine Farmer* says: "Mosquitoes love beef-blood better than they do any that flows in the veins of human kind. Just put a couple of generous pieces of beef on plates near your bed at night, and you will sleep untroubled by those pests. In the mornings you will find them full and stupid with beef-blood, and the meat sucked as dry as a cork.

August 1, 1865

❀

To Cure Piles - Ira F. Seudder writes in the *Rural*: "Wild turnips will cure the piles. Prevention is better than cure. Let the afflicted carry it in their pockets. A very simple thing will make a man sick, why not a simple thing cure him ?"

August 15, 1865

❀

Smoke For The Cure of Wounds - A correspondent of the *Albany Country Gentleman* recommends smoke as a curative agent for wounds in men and animals. He says: "I cut my foot with an axe. The lady of the house, seizing the foot while it was yet bleeding freely, held it over a pan containing smoking tag locks (ragged lock of wool on sheep). In a few minutes the bleeding stopped, the smoke was removed and a bandage applied to protect it from accidental blows. The wound never suppurated, and consequently never pained me. I have seen the remedy tried in many similar cases, and always with the same result. Let the reader bear in mind that no liniment or salve, drawing or healing, should be applied. You have merely to smoke the wound well and nature will do the rest."

September 1, 1865

❀

Our Eyes - Reading with the gas light before you is another cause of weak eyes. The light should always hang quite high and behind you, and be allowed to hang over the shoulder. If convenient it should be over the left shoulder. If using kerosene, it is best to employ the lamps which hang on the wall. Neither should you read with your face toward the window. Reading by twilight is dangerous. Gradually accommodating itself to the receding twilight, the eye is unconsciously strained. I have seen more than

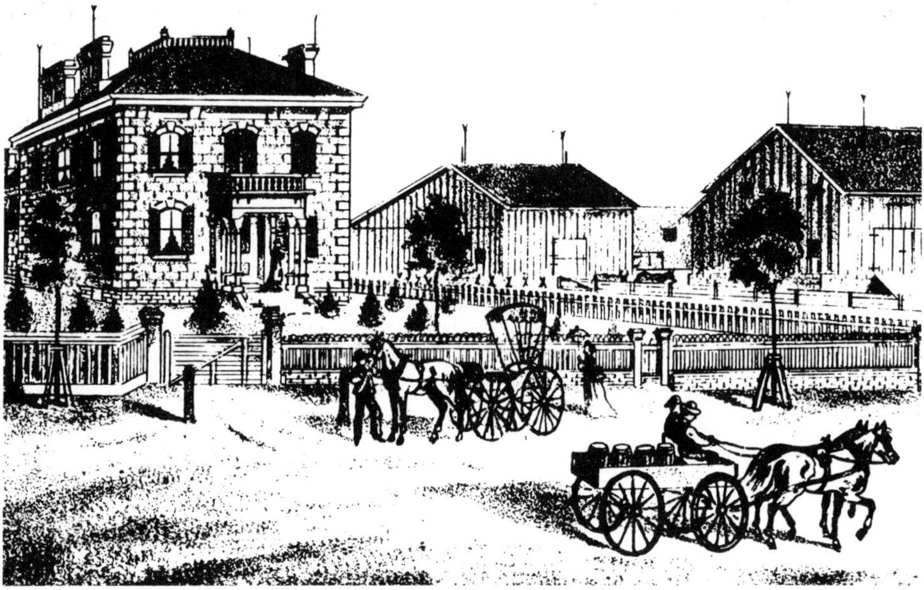

one case of grave disease of the eye, produced by an undue effort to use the vision too long at twilight. Avoid reading by artificial light when you can. We read too much. We read as we eat—pell-mell, hotichity-potch; no mastication, no digestion. If, as a people, we read less we might know more.

The newspapers have much to answer for in the way of small type and imperfect printing. I would cheerfully give two hundred dollars a year to support a newspaper which would give us, morning and evening, a half column of the really reliable news, instead of fifteen columns of diluted speculations and tricky canards, the reading of which hurts our eyes and wastes our precious time.

November 15, 1865

❀

Girls, Beware! - Girls, beware of transient young men. Never suffer the addresses of a stranger. Recollect that one good farmer's boy, or industrious mechanic, is worth all the floating fops in the world. The allurements of a dandy Jack, with a gold chain round his neck, a walking stick in his paw, a three-penny cigar in his mouth, or some honest tailor's coat on his back, and a brainless, though fancy skull, never can make up the loss of a good father's home, and a good mother's counsel, and the society of brothers and sisters; their affections last, while that of such a young man is lost in the wane of the honeymoon. 'Tis true.

November 15, 1865

Cure For Cholera - Dr. Chapman publishes a pamphlet to show that in the application of ice to the spine he has found a powerful remedy for cholera, and the slighter complaint of diarrhoea. He has only had the chance of trying his theoretic remedy on one case of cholera, and that, though it had all the worst symptoms, was probably a severe case of English rather than genuine Asiatic cholera. However, in that case it proved to be exceedingly effective in subduing all the more dangerous symptoms.

November 15, 1865

❀

Why Children Die - The reason why children die is because they are not taken care of. From the day of their birth they are stuffed with food, choked with physic, suffocated in hot rooms, steamed in bed clothes. So much for indoors. When permitted to breathe a breath of air once a week in summer, and once or twice during the cold months, only the nose is permitted to peer into daylight. A little later they are sent out without no clothes at all, as to the parts of the body which need most protection. Bare legs, bare arms, bare necks, girted middles, with an inverted umbrella to collect the air and chill the other parts of the body. A stout, strong man goes out on a cold day with gloves and overcoat, woollen stockings, and thick double-soled boots. The same day a child of three years old, an infant in flesh and blood, and bone and constitution goes out with soles as thin as paper, cotton socks, legs uncovered to the knees, neck bare; an exposure which would disable the nurse, kill the mother in a fortnight, and make the father an invalid for weeks. And why? To harden them to a mode of dress which they are never expected to practise. To accustom them to exposure, which a dozen years later would be considered downright foolish. To rear children thus for the slaughter pen, and then lay it to Heaven, is too bad.

March 15, 1866

❀

Coffee As A Disinfectant - We learn from *The Farmer* that Dr. Barbier affirms that ground coffee possesses some remarkable properties as a disinfectant. In several cases where he had to make post-mortem examinations of bodies under very disagreeable circumstances, he found that a handful of coffee strewn over the body and about the room quite overcame any bad odour.

May 15, 1866

Petroleum For Asthma - A correspondent of the *Country Gentleman* writes in that journal: "I have a son, six years old, that had the asthma in the most distressing form for three or four months, when he was one or two years old. We tried everything we could hear of without getting relief, till we were told to rub his neck and breast with petroleum, and we used it both crude and refined, experiencing very speedy relief and a final and permanent cure; for he has not since had a return of it, and is now a very healthy child."

May 15, 1866

❀

Hair-wash For Dandruff - The *Scientific American* gives the following recipe: Take one pint of alcohol and a tablespoonful of castor oil, mix them together in a bottle by shaking them well for a few minutes, then scent it with a few drops of lavender. Alcohol dissolves castor oil, like gum camphor, leaving the liquid or wash quite clear. It does not seem to dissolve any other unctuous oil so perfectly, hence no other is equally good for this purpose.

June 1, 1866

❀

Facts Worth Remembering - "Cosmo", in the Philadelphia *Saturday Evening Post*, gives the following facts worth remembering:

1. It is worth while, for all farmers everywhere, to remember that thorough culture is better than three mortgages on their farm.
2. That an offensive war against weeds, is five times less expensive than a defensive one.
3. That good fences always pay better than law suits with neighbours.
4. That hay is a great deal cheaper made in the summer, than purchased in the winter.
5. That a horse who lays his ears back and looks lightning when any one approaches him, is vicious. Don't buy him.
6. That scrimping the feed of fatting hogs, is a waste of grain.
7. That over-fed fowls won't lay eggs.
8. That educating children is money lent at a hundred percent.
9. That one evening spent at home in study, is more profitable than ten lounging about country taverns.

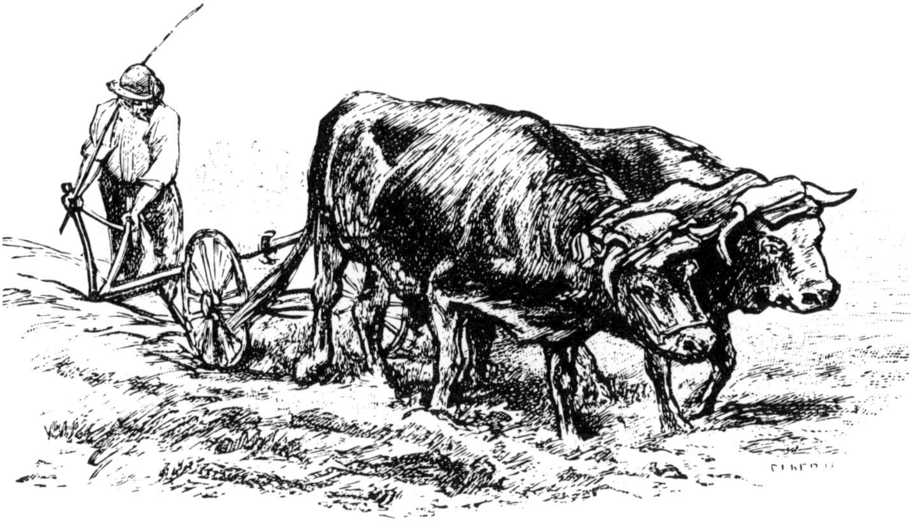

10. That cows should always be milked regularly and clean.

11. That it is the duty of every man to take some good, reliable, entertaining paper, and pay for it promptly of course.

July 2, 1866

❀

Hay Fever - A correspondent of *The Times* suggests an instant and sensible relief to this complaint—bathing the nostrils and closed eyes with spirits of camphor and warm water.

July 16, 1866

❀

Children's Sleeping Rooms - We clip the following judicious observations from the *Family Herald*: "Most parents, before retiring to rest, make it a duty to visit the sleeping-rooms of their children. They do so in order to be satisfied that the lights are extinguished, and that no danger is threatening their little ones. But if they leave the room with closed windows and doors, they shut in as great an enemy as fire, although his ravages may not be so readily detected. Poison is there, slow but deadly. Morning after morning do many little children wake weary, fretful and oppressed. 'What can it mean?' 'What can it be?' the mother cries. In despair she has recourse to medicine. The constitution becomes enfeebled, and the child gets worse. The cause, perhaps, is never traced to over-crowded sleeping rooms, without proper air; but is, nevertheless, the right one. An intelligent mother, having acquainted herself with the principles of ventilation, will not retire to her own room for the night without having provided sufficiency of air for her children, in the same manner that she provides and regulates their nightcovering, or any other requisite for refreshing slumber.

October 15, 1866

❀

To Avoid Cholera (sensible advice) - An American paper, among other suggestions which will enable a person to avoid the cholera, says: "Endeavour, if possible, to keep a clear conscience, and two or three clean shirts. Rise with the lark, but avoid larks in the evening. Be above ground in all your dwellings, and above board in all your dealings. Love your neighbour as yourself, but don't have too many in the same house with you."

June 15, 1867

❀

Hints To Farmers' Daughters - To the Editor of The *Canada Farmer*:

Sir, - In your issue of June the first, I read a communication entitled "Hints to Farmers' Daughters;" and, as I consider it a misrepresentation of our farmers' daughters, I am induced to write a brief reply, so that the public may obtain both sides of the question.

I can see a great distinction between city and country girls, and I must say that city girls are unfit for the wives of farmers, on account of their ignorance of country work in general; but every country girl should know how to milk, spin, bake etc. Farmers' daughters should be industrious, economical housekeepers, should understand all the etceteras of milk, butter, cheese, spinning, sewing, etc; and so should every country girl, whether her father is a blacksmith, weaver or whatever his calling may be. They can all get a suitable education to fit them for model farmers' wives, so that there will be an abundance of rosy girls to help the young farmer along, as well as a choice for every old bachelor who lives in his lonely hall; or for any farmer who doesn't want a woman who can play the piano, but one who can only make cheese, talk cheese, and eat cheese. Then there will be fitting companions for those who, by their education, want a companion they can converse with—who, while she makes the best of everything, can talk on the topics of the day, and has a mind that thirsts for knowledge. So cheer up, farmers; there are trimmings for every kind of cloth. Make yourselves worthy of the girls, and there is no danger of anybody rivalling you in winning that inestimable treasure, a good farmer's daughter.

July 15, 1867

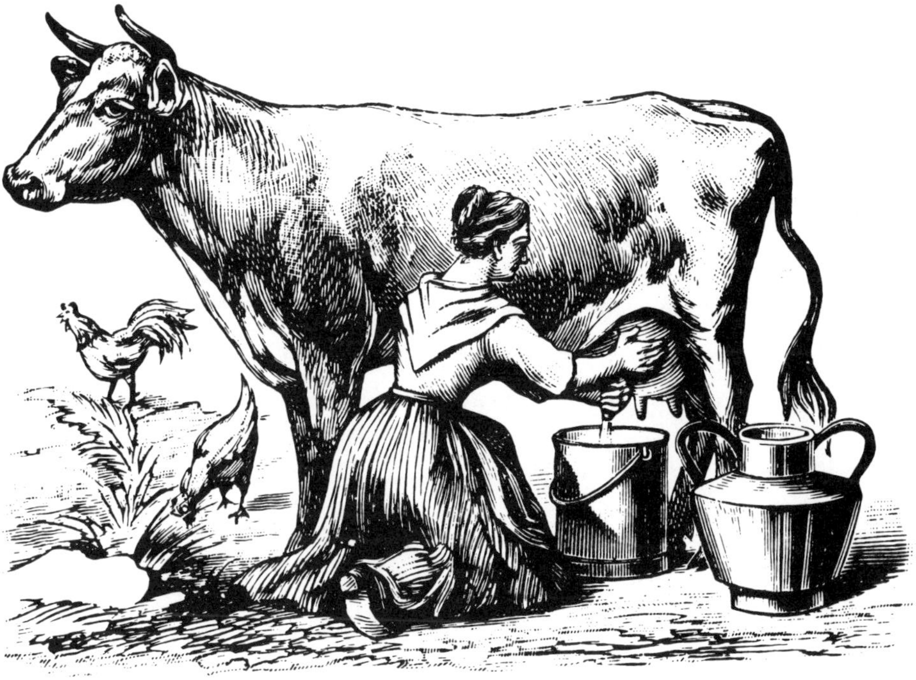

A Mistake - A good lady who had two children sick with measles, wrote to a friend for the best remedy. The friend has just received a note from another lady, inquiring the way to pickle cucumbers. In the confusion, the lady who inquired about the pickles received the remedy for the measles, and the anxious mother of the sick children, with horror read the following. "Scald them three or four times in very hot vinegar, and sprinkle them with salt, and in a very few days they will be cured."

August 15, 1867

❀

Sleeping In Cold Room - *Hall's Journal of Health* says that cold bed-chambers always imperil health, and invite fatal disease. Robust persons may safely sleep in a temperature of forty degrees, or under, but the old, the infant, and the frail, should never sleep in a room where the atmosphere is much under fifty degrees Fahrenheit.

Many persons wake up in the morning with inflammation of the lungs who went to bed well, and are surprised that this should be the case. The cause may often be found in sleeping in a room the window of which has been foolishly hoisted for ventilation. The water-cure journals of the country have done an incalculable injury by the blind and indiscriminate advice of hoisting the window at night.

The rule should be everywhere during the part of the year when fires are kept burning, to avoid hoisting outside windows. It is safer, and better to leave the chamber-door open, as also the fireplace—then there is a draft up the chimney, while the room is not so likely to become cold. If there is some fire in the room all night, the window may be opened an inch. It is better to sleep in a bad air all night with a temperature over fifty, than in a pure air with a temperature under forty. The bad air may sicken you, but cannot kill you; the cold air can, and does kill very often.

December 30, 1873

❀

Country Physicians - "Why should not Country Physicians study veterinary practice so that they could give advice in regard to the troubles of farm stock?" The *American Agriculturist* thinks it would be of immense advantage to farmers if such a thing could be brought about, and that it would tend to rid the country of a host of quacks and "cow-doctors," so called, who are ignorant of what they profess, and often inflict much needless suffering upon animals. We agree with our contemporary on this point. Relieving the sufferings of the animals subjected to us is a mission only less noble than that of healing the "Lord of Creation" himself. Many a country physician, from motives of humanity alone, would prescribe for sick horses and cattle were it not that he would lose caste if he were to lift a finger to save a poor brute from agony. And many struggling young doctors, who are now eking out their existence in shabby gentility and enforced idleness, could be placed at once in comfortable circumstances if they were permitted to avail themselves of practice within easy reach. Away, say we, with the ridiculous nonsense that will allow animals to suffer, frauds to flourish, and competent men to starve, just to gratify the requirements of overstrained professional etiquette.

May 15, 1875

Patent Medicines

The proliferation of nostrums, patent or propriety medicines was a major social and economic phenomenon at the end of the 19th century. In a significant sense, this development can be related to the nature of self-help medicine, in that there still remained a practical public scepticism of the medical profession and its costs (unless one was forced to use them in cases of major life threatening sickness), and an ingrained belief and practice that individuals and families could and should be able to treat their own ailments.

"Patent" medicines (although formal patents were not required or even normally obtained) were easily available by mail order and at drug stores or local general stores. Some were produced and distributed by "quacks," while others emerged from more established and therefore more "reputable" manufacturers. The growth and increased availability of newspapers containing extensive advertising reinforced the obvious economic motive of the "patent" proprietors. Were individuals merely being gullible in their apparent willingness to believe in or try any commercial nostrum which claimed to cure an almost endless list of ailments? Did they "work?" Perhaps some did. Others may have succeeded merely by their placebo effect—others not at all. Were they bought and used? Yes, extensively, by the general population, whether rich or poor.

Dr. R. V. Pierce, founder of the "World's Dispensary Medical Association," operated the Invalids' Hotel and Surgical Institute in Buffalo, New York, and produced *The People's Common Sense Medical Advisor in Plain English; or Medicine Simplified*. It was first published in 1875, and over the next sixty years was to be reprinted one hundred times. In the 88th edition (1921), a wide variety of medicines were advertised which could be obtained by mail "on receipt of the price quoted" from his Laboratory in Buffalo or from Bridgeburg, Ontario. Dr. Pierce's Family Medicines, which were advertised in this book, included:

- Golden Medical Discovery - invigorates and cleanses the whole system
- Favourite Prescription - for female weakness, barrenness, morning sickness, hysteria, nervousness
- Anuric Tablets - kidney, bladder, backache

- Irontic Tablets - if the blood is impoverished, we feel nervous, sleepless, "fidgety"
- Chill Tonic Pills - a remarkable remedy for malaria
- Pleasant Pellets - bilious and sick headache, dizziness, constipation, indigestion
- Catarrh Tablets - removes mucous and purulent deposits
- Extract of Smart-Weed - internally for cramps, diarrhoea, colic; externally for sprains, bruises, neuralgia, pain in the back

In addition, the book contained a large number of glowing personal endorsements, together with a photograph of the cured sufferer which appeared under such captions as: "indigestion and torpid liver cured by special home-treatment," "a remarkable effect of one bottle," "used in family for thirty years with excellent results" and "saved from the knife."

The Dr. A. W. Chase Medicine Company of Toronto and Buffalo was another major producer and distributor of patent medicines, which was initially established in Ann Arbor, Michigan following Dr. Chase's publication of his famous *Dr. Chase's Recipes or Information for Everybody* (1863, 12th edition). The company's fifty-two page calendar and almanac for 1914 contained a large number of advertising captions followed by glowing testimonials to the wonderful cures obtained: "Was operated on, wound did not heal," "Doctor puzzled, gave him up," "Remarkable cure of most serious case," "Was pale and thin, skin was yellow." The company's large range of Dr. Chase's remedies included Ointment, Liver Cure, Catarrh Powder, Syrup of Linseed and Turpentine, Kidney-Liver Pills, Nerve Food and Backache Plaster. Indeed, as the publication noted, the readers should: "Keep well by having Dr. Chase your family doctor." Thus the company continued even though he had died in 1885.

A particularly interesting participant in "the golden age of patent medicine" in the decades before World War I was the Dr. William's Medicine Company, operated by the G. T. Fulford Company with its production and distribution of Pink Pills for Pale People. George Taylor Fulford (1852-1905) was an entrepreneur and politician who was born in Brockville, Canada West. In 1887, having identified a growing market for self-help medical products, he set up his own patent medicine company. In the late 19th century the emergence of the popular press, an improved and relatively inexpensive transportation system based on the railroads and an expanding manufacturing technology had set the stage for the

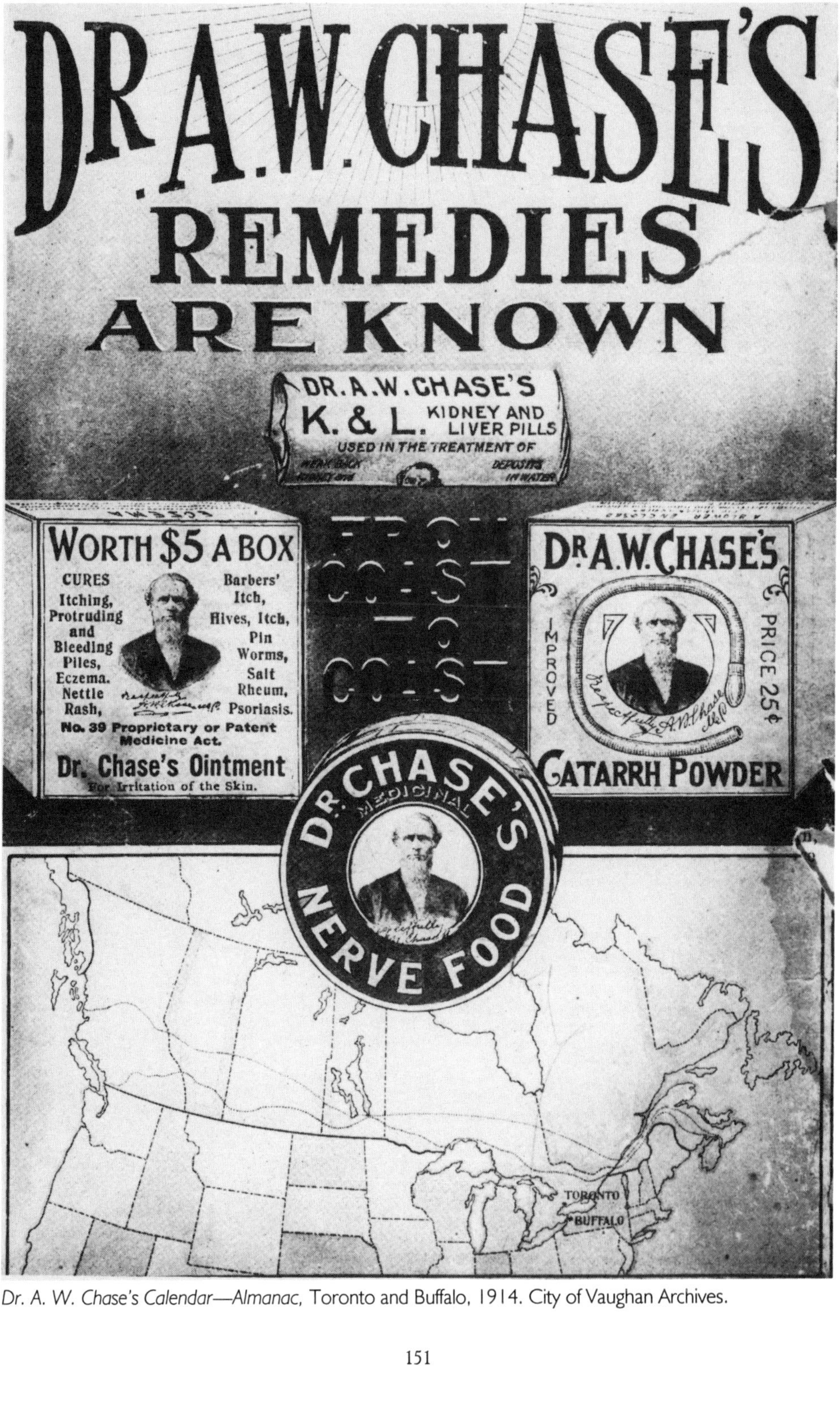

Dr. A. W. Chase's Calendar—Almanac, Toronto and Buffalo, 1914. City of Vaughan Archives.

patent medicine phenomenon. Fulford's shrewd marketing skills and willingness to advertise extensively soon brought positive results. By the early 20th century, with his Pink Pills selling for 50¢ a box or six boxes for $2.50, yearly consumption in Canada was estimated at one million boxes.

By this time, branches of the company had been established as far away as London, Paris, Singapore, Rio de Janeiro, and Cape Town. In 1900, Fulford was appointed to the Canadian Senate by Sir Wilfrid Laurier, after having reputedly (if not appropriately) made a donation of $5,000 to the Liberal Party. At his death in 1905, his various interests were valued at almost $5 million. As a footnote, Canadian legislation which was passed in 1909 required patent medicine companies to list the ingredients in their products and attempted to control their often bizarre advertising claims.

To give an example of the role of newspapers in the patent medicine era, the April 4, 1884 edition of the *Woodstock Sentinel-Review* (Woodstock, Ontario) carried the following paid advertisements:

- *Burdock Blood Bitters* - will cure or relieve biliousness, jaundice, headache, fluttering of the heart, dryness of the skin, etc.
- *Dr. E. C. West's Nerve and Brain Treatment* - a guaranteed specific for hysteria, convulsions, mental depression, softening of the brain, premature old age, loss of power in either sex, etc.
- *Hagyard's Yellow Oil* - cures rheumatism.
- *Freeman's Worm Powders* - a safe, sure and effectual destroyer of worms in children or adults.
- *Kidney-Wort* - the sure cure for kidney diseases, liver complaints, constipation, piles and blood diseases.
- *Sulphur and Iron Bitters* - will give sleep, sound and refreshing in due season; strengthens feeble women and makes puny children strong; will infuse with new life the weakest invalid.
- *Lyman's Universal Pain Reliever* - for frost bite, cramps, rheumatism, neuralgic affections, and toothache, full directions with each bottle ($2.00).

Indeed the list of such products and their overblown claims is almost limitless. The fifty years prior to WWI comprised the golden age of "patent" medicines. The following editorial from The *Canada Farmer*, May 15, 1869 comments, albeit in a negative way, on this phenomenon:

> "But on the whole, perhaps the greatest evil from which they suffer is the great faith they have in the quack nostrums and patent medicines so largely advertised in every country paper. Every country store contains a large stock of these worthless rubbish, and we are told that were it not for the demand for patent medicines among country people, their manufacture would have to be abandoned, instead of, as now, being the stepping stone on which many an illiterate quack has built up a colossal fortune out of the hard-won earnings of industrious farmers.
>
> Perhaps most of these patent medicines are not of themselves poisonously injurious, but at the best they are utterly useless for any good purposes, and their virtues exist only in the advertisements of their proprietors and the imaginations of those who read them. They are, as a general rule, purposely made of such materials as have both a stimulating and soothing effect on the system, and so excite a desire for their continued use when once they have been taken, alcohol and opium being the base and principal ingredients in most of them; and their use, though it may seemingly result in relief from an imaginary complaint, ultimately deranges first the digestive powers, and soon the whole bodily frame, causing disease and general ill-health.
>
> With good, wholesome, well-cooked food; enough work in the open air to sharpen the appetite and fully exercise the body, followed by balmy sleep, "nature's sweet restorer," the farmer may say, "Throw physic to the dogs, I'll none of it."

18 FAMILY RECEIPT BOOK.

DARLEY'S ARABIAN OIL!

FOR HORSES AND CATTLE,

AND

UNIVERSAL FAMILY LINIMENT.

A NEVER-FAILING REMEDY.

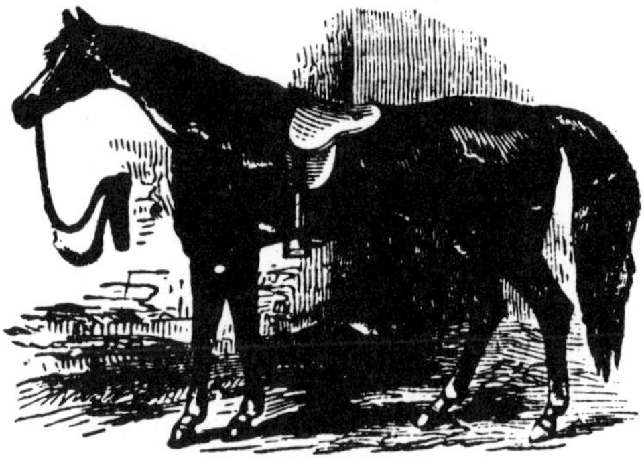

This valuable preparation combines all the medicinal virtues of those articles which long experience has proved to possess the most safe and efficient properties for the cure of

Flesh Wounds, Sprains, Bruises,
Galls of all kinds, Cracked Heels,
Ring Bone, Spavins,
Windgalls, Callous,
Fistula, Sweeney,
External Poisons,
Scratches or Grease,
Strains, Lameness,
Mange, Whitlows, Corns,
Sand Cracks, Foundered Feet,
Horn Distemper,
Swelling,
Rheumatism, Cramps,
Chilblains,
Caked Breasts, Boils,
Bites of Animals,
Weakness of the Joints,
Contraction of Muscles,
Burns and Scalds,
Frost Bites,
Painful Nervous Affections,
Chapped Hands,
Tumors,
Old Sores,

AND MANY OTHER DISEASES WHICH MAN AND BEAST ARE SUBJECT TO.

Family Receipt Book, 1869, Metropolitan Toronto Reference Library

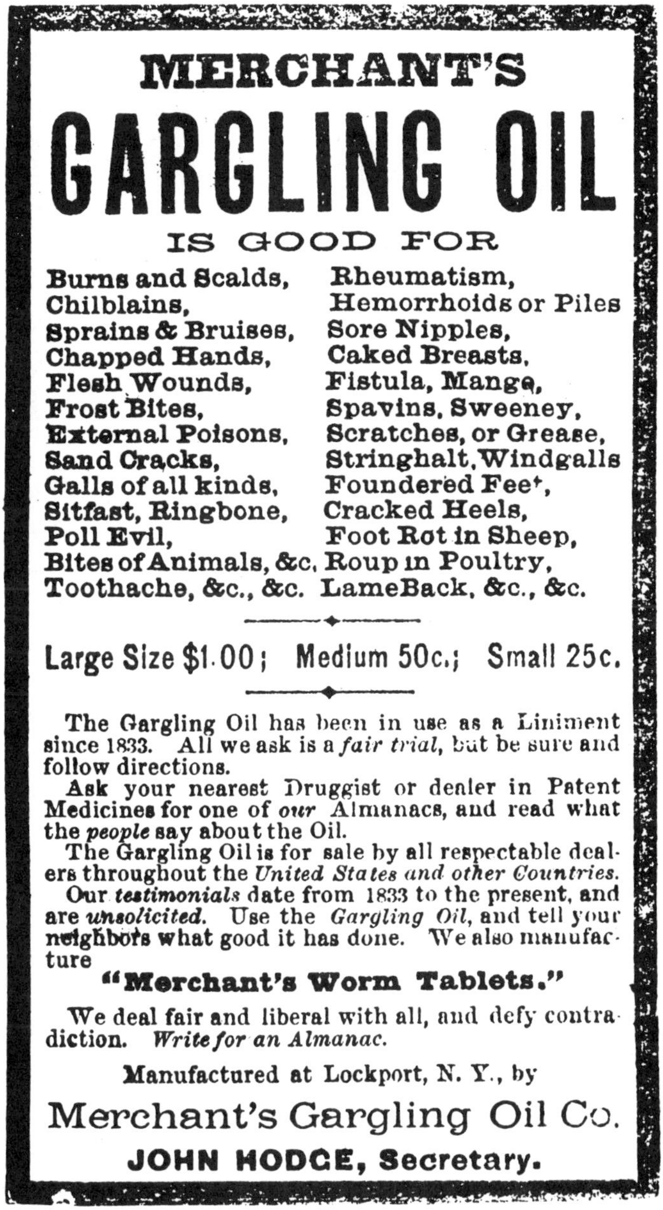

The *Canada Farmer*, October 15, 1872

HAGYARD'S

YELLOW OIL

Greatest Cure in the World.
Give it One Trial.

This Oil is the only remedy for the cure of

Rheumatism, Neuralgia, Lumbago, Spinal and Bronchial Complaints, Deafness, Head-Ache, Ear-Ache, Cramps, Sprains, Bruises, Stiff Joints, Galls, Swelled Hands, Sore Nipples, Stiff Neck, Chilblains,

Tetter, Frost Bites, Chapped Hands, Cuts, Wounds, Sore Throat, Stings of Insects, Shortness of Breath, or any Diseases that are painful and sore.

It is the only article ever brought before the public that will do its work perfectly, and has been used by thousands and pronounced to be the best remedy for relieving pain ever discovered.

The Cheapest Medicine Ever Made for Internal and External Use.

Guide Book and Atlas of Muskoka and Parry Sound Districts, Toronto, 1879

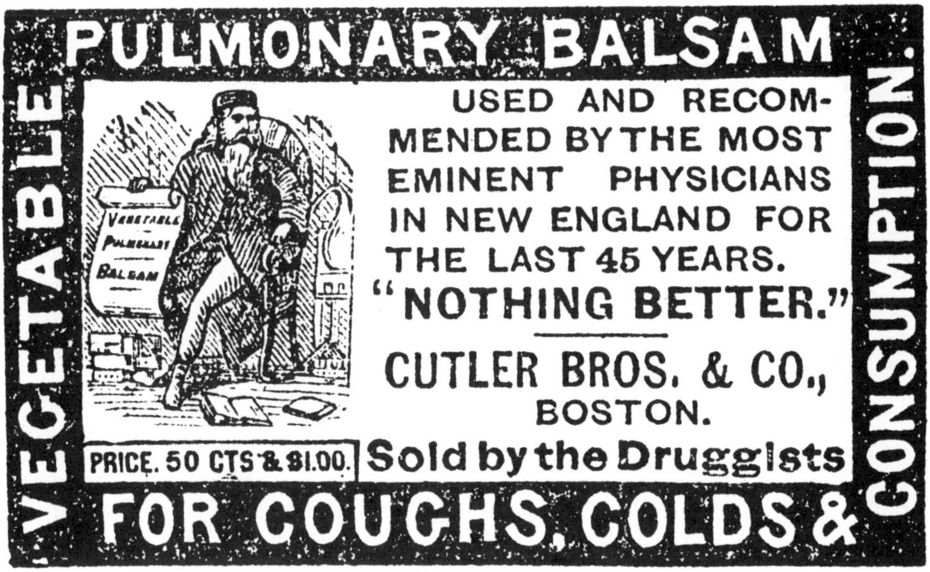

The *Canada Farmer*, March 25, 1872

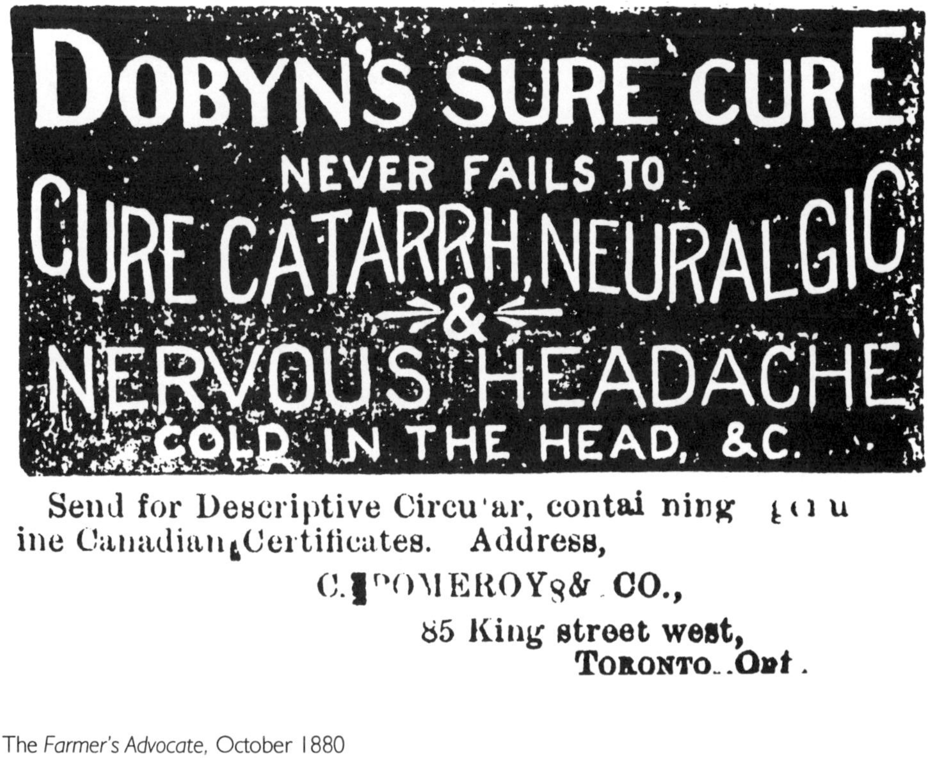

The *Farmer's Advocate*, October 1880

Burdock Blood Bitters

Cures Billiousness, Jaundice Dyspepsia, Constipation, Nervous and General Debility, Headache, Rheumatism, Scrofula, Dropsy, Female Complaints, Erysipelas, Salt Rheum, and every species of Chronic Disease arising from Disordered Liver Kidneys, Stomach Bowels or Blood.

THE BEST BLOOD PURIFYING TONIC IN THE WORLD.

ITS VIRTUES ACKNOWLEDGED.

MR. R. C. BALMER OAKVILLE, Nov. 16, 1880.

Dear Sir.—It affords me unqualified pleasure to bear testimony to the benefit I have experienced from using Burdock Blood Bitters. For several years I have suffered from oft-recurring billious Headaches, Dyspepsia, and complaints peculiar to my sex, which now I am entirely relieved from, if not cured, by using only about half a bottle of the Bitters. I now beg to return you my sincere thanks for recommending to me such a valuable medicine.

I remain, yours sincerely, MRS. IRA MULLHOLDAND.

Mother Hubbard's Cupboard or *Canadian Cookbook*, Hamilton, Ontario: G.C. Briggs, 1881

ST. JACOBS OIL

TRADE MARK

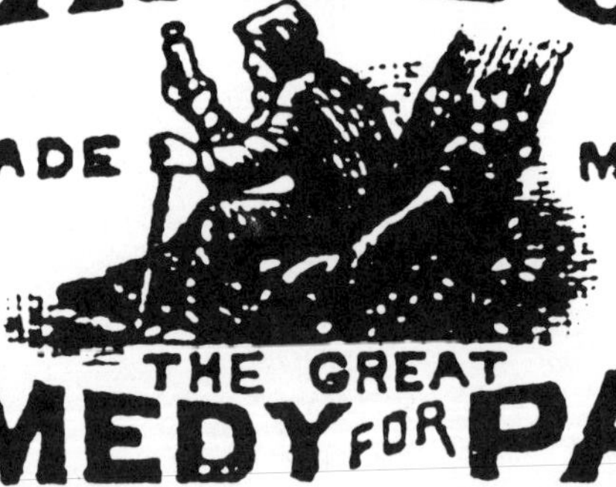

THE GREAT REMEDY FOR PAIN

CURES—Rheumatism, Neuralgia, Sciatica, Lumbago, Backache, Headache, Toothache, Sore Throat, Burns, Scalds, Swellings, Frostbites, Sprains, Bruises, Wounds.

The Charles A. Vogeler Company, Brockville, Ont., 1889-?, CIHM 64939

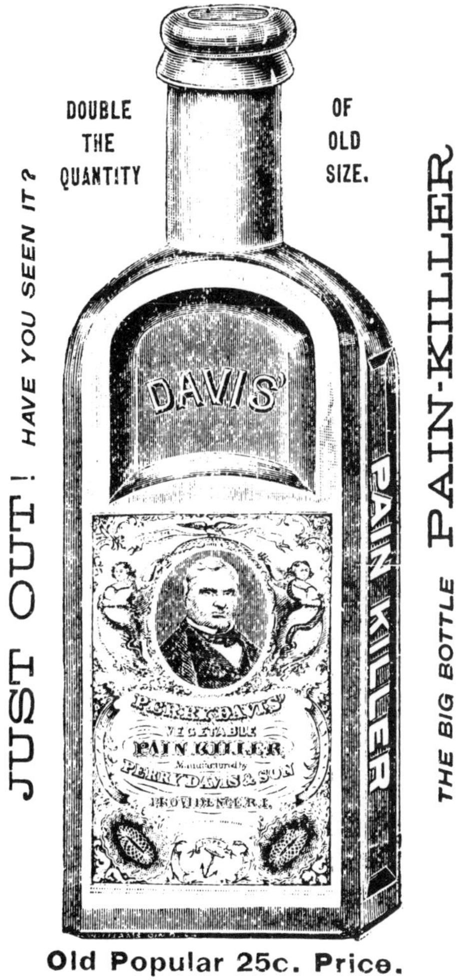

Metropolitan Toronto Library, 89D2, 189-

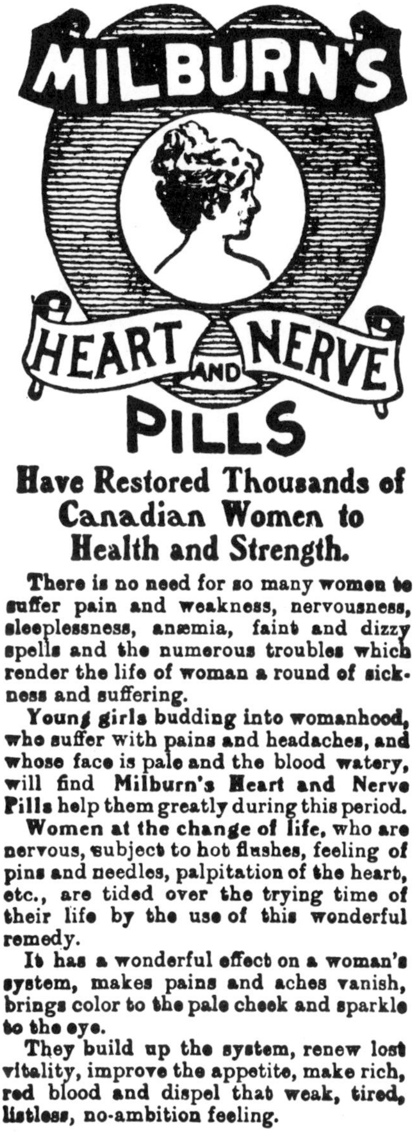

The *Farmer's Advocate*, July 27, 1905

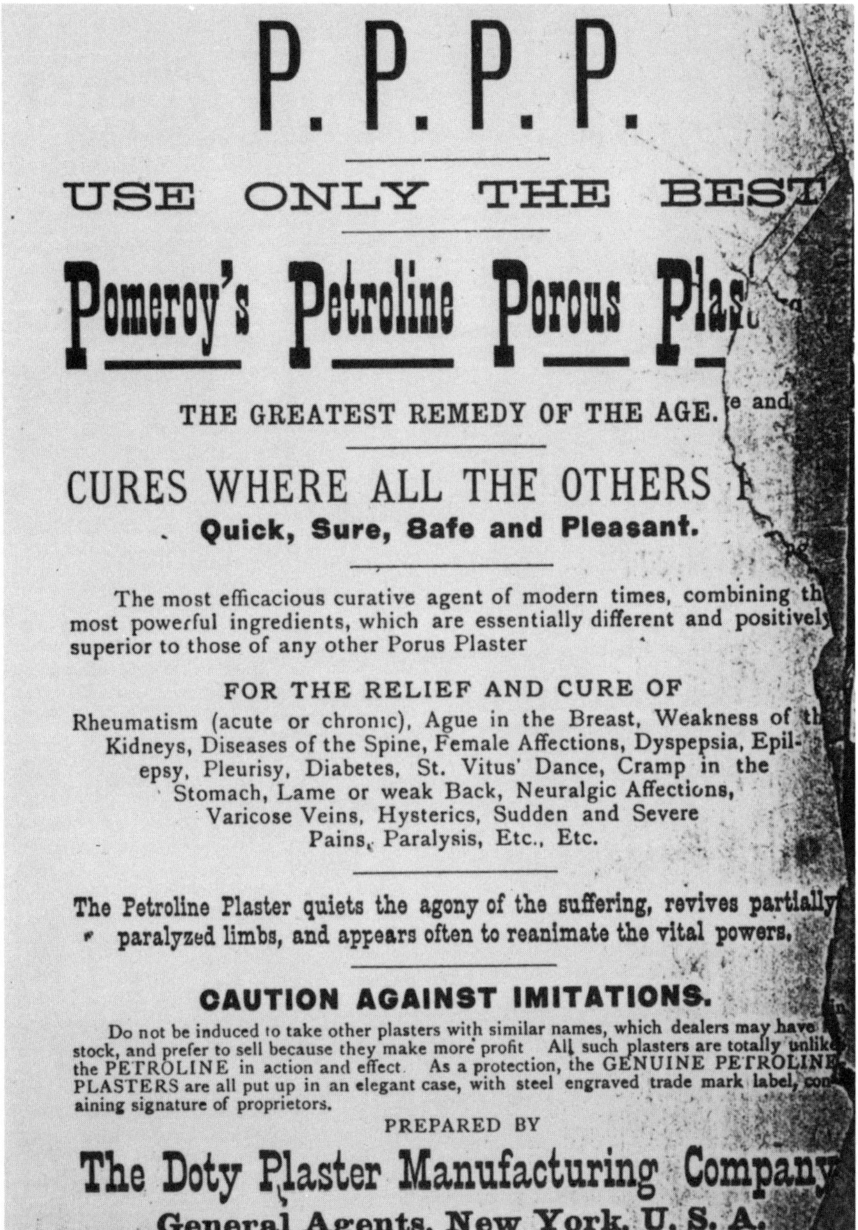

Mother Hubbard's Cupboard or *Canadian Cookbook*, Hamilton, Ontario: G.C. Briggs, 1881

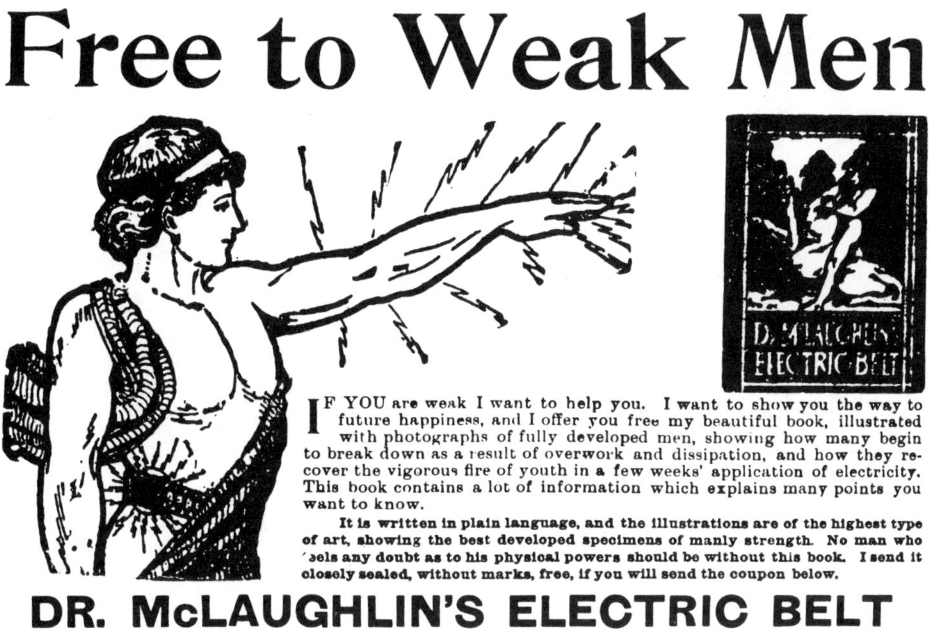

The *Farmer's Advocate*, July 6, 1905

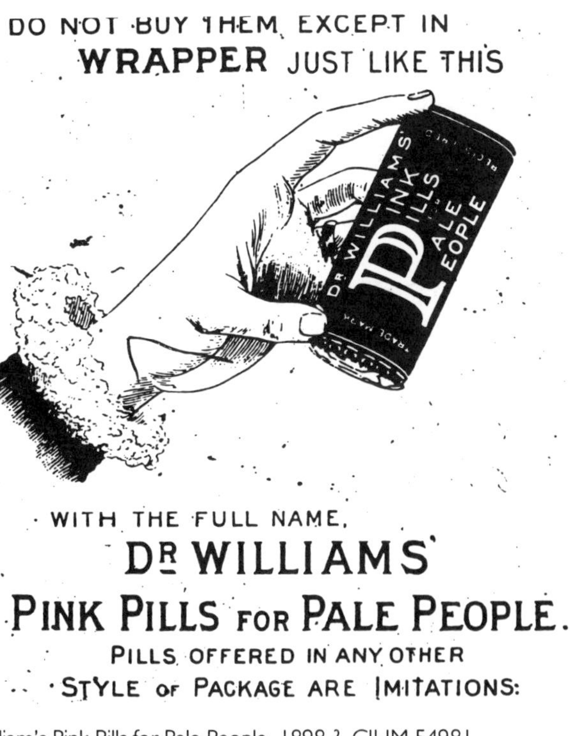

Dr. William's Pink Pills for Pale People, 1898-?, CIHM 54981

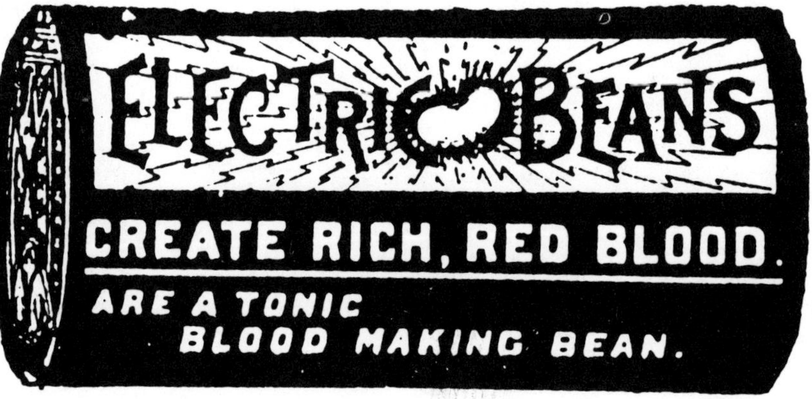

ELECTRIC BEANS

Stand supreme as a Blood and Nerve Tonic.

They are unequalled for Billiousness, Sick Headache, Constipation, Heart Palpitation, Indigestion and Anæmia.

Those who are in a position to know what is best use "ELECTRIC BEANS."

Write for Free Sample

50c. a Box at all Dealers or upon receipt of price, from

THE ELECTRIC BEAN CHEMICAL CO. Ltd.
OTTAWA.

The *Farmer's Advocate*, July 14, 1910

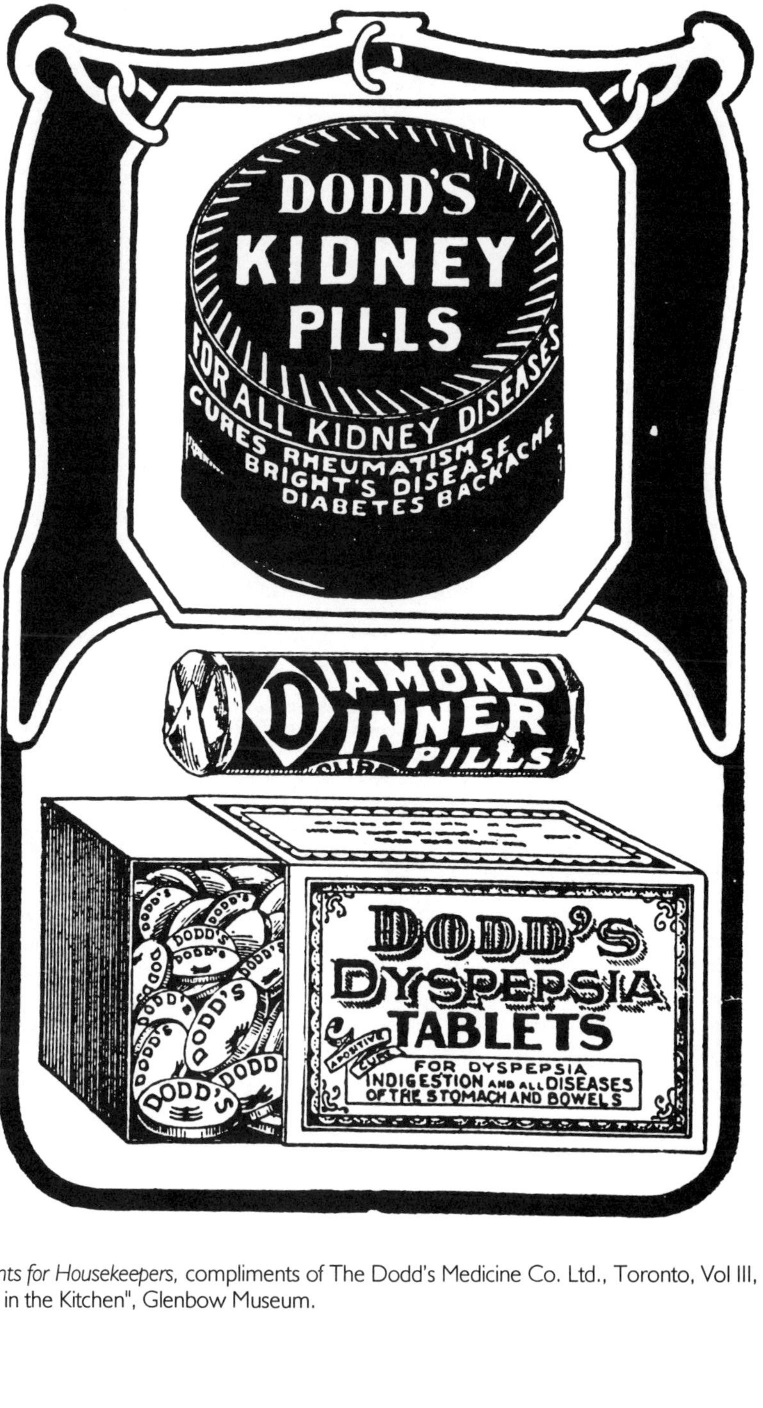

Helpful Hints for Housekeepers, compliments of The Dodd's Medicine Co. Ltd., Toronto, Vol III, 1913, "Hang Me in the Kitchen", Glenbow Museum.

Like his famous Receipt Book Dr. Chase's Medicines are always reliable 11

Worn Out by Housework

Tired out—unable to rest or sleep—easily irritated and excited—depressed and discouraged

Housework is monotonous and tiresome, the more tiresome because it is so monotonous. Doing the same thing over and over again, day in and day out, is what breaks down the nervous system.

And housework is hard work. Let any man do a Monday's washing or a Friday's sweeping, in addition to the other duties which crowd themselves into every day; and then asked him if he is tired.

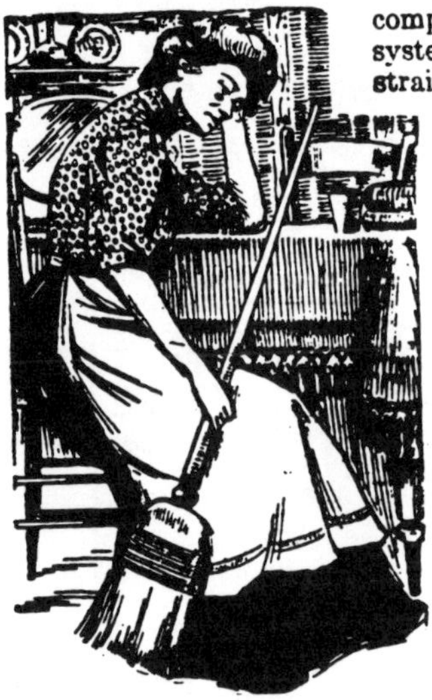

But most women work away without murmur or complaint, so long as health is good. It is only when the system breaks down under constant and monotonous strain that life becomes well-nigh unbearable.

With the blood thin and watery, the nerves become feeble and starved, and cry out with terrible neuralgic headaches, or sciatic rheumatism, or weakness which almost equals helplessness.

With the delicate nerves jangled out of tune, little things annoy and irritate one; slight overexertion or excitement brings sleepless nights, with dark forebodings for the future. In some cases irritability reaches such a pitch as to make one think of insanity.

What is to be done? A trip abroad or a long rest in a sanitarium? For the rich this is possible, but the great majority of mothers must fight it out in their own homes, and for them there is nothing like Dr. Chase's Nerve Food.

Gentle and natural in its upbuilding influence on the system, this great food cure seems to be admirably suited to the delicate nervous system of women.

Each dose goes to form a certain amount of pure, rich blood. This in turn nourishes the feeble, wasted nerve cells back to health and vigor, and instils new energy and strength into every part of the body.

Dr. A. W. Chasé's Calendar—Almanac, Toronto and Buffalo, 1914, City of Vaughan Archives

Primitive Physic ~ John Wesley

John Wesley (1703-1791), the founder of Methodism, was born in Lincolnshire, England. He initially took priestly orders in the Church of England but, following a three-year stay in the American Colonies in 1738, "through the influence of the Moravians, he acquired a conviction that Christ had a special concern for him, directly communicated and implemented, and that trust in Christ was adequate for his soul's salvation."[1] His constant travels and preachings soon led to the establishment of Methodist Societies in Britain and America, which then followed the United Empire Loyalists and subsequent immigrants into Canada.

Wesley's religious and humanitarian beliefs led him to focus on the condition of the poor and disadvantaged, of which there were many. In 1747, he published *Primitive Physick: or, An Easy and Natural Method of Curing Most Diseases.* By 1828, there were thirty-two London editions, and seven editions were published in the United States between 1764 and 1839. Wesley had read widely on the subject of medical treatments and believed in the critical values of experience and common sense. He was strongly opposed to the "Herculean medicines" of opium, quinine, and quicksilver, commonly used by the medical profession of the period. His aim was:

> "to set down cheap, safe and easy medicines; easy to be known, easy to be procured, and easy to be applied by plain unlettered men—to recommend to men of plain unbiased reason such remedies as air, water, milk, whey, honey, treacle, salt, vinegar and common English herbs, with a few foreign medicines almost equally cheap, safe, and common. And this I have done on that principle whereby I desire to be governed in all my actions, 'Whatsoever ye would that men should do unto you, the same do unto them'."[2]

While at Oxford, Wesley had been greatly impressed by Dr. Cheyne's *Book on Health and Long Life* which emphasized the importance of temperance, exercises, and a common sense diet. Thus Wesley began his book by giving the following plain easy rules, chiefly transcribed from Dr. Cheyne, "for the sake of those who desire, through the blessing of God, to retain the health which they have recovered."

Plain Easy Rules:

1. a. The air we breathe is of great consequence to our health. Those who have been long abroad in easterly or northerly winds should drink some thin and warm liquor going to bed, or a draught of toast and water.

   b. Tender people should have those who lie with them, or are much about them, sound, sweet, and healthy.

   c. Every one that would preserve health should be as clean and sweet as possible in their houses, clothes, and furniture.

2. a. The great rule of eating and drinking is to suit the quality and quantity of the food to the strength of the digestion; to take always such a sort and such a measure of food as sits light and easy on the stomach.

   b. All pickled, or smoked, or salted, and all high-seasoned, food is unwholesome.

   c. Nothing conduces more to health than abstinence and plain food, with due labour.

   d. For studious persons, about eight ounces of animal food, and twelve of vegetable, in twenty-four hours, is sufficient.

   e. Water is the wholesomest of all drinks; it quickens the appetite, and strengthens the digestion most.

   f. Strong, and more especially spirituous liquors, are a certain, though slow, poison.

   g. Experience shews there is very seldom any danger in leaving them off all at once.

   h. Strong liquors do not prevent the mischiefs of a surfeit, nor carry it off so safely as water.

   i. Malt liquors, except clear small beer, or small ale of due age, are extremely hurtful to tender persons.

   j. Coffee and tea are extremely hurtful to persons who have weak nerves.

3. a. Tender persons should eat very light suppers, and that two or three hours before going to bed.

b. They ought constantly to go to bed about nine, and rise at four or five.

4. a. A due degree of exercise is indispensably necessary to health and long life.

b. Walking is the best exercise for those who are able to bear it; riding for those who are not. The open air, when the weather is fair, contributes much to the benefit of exercise.

c. We may strengthen any weak part of the body by constant exercise. Thus the lungs may be strengthened by loud speaking, or walking up an easy ascent; the digestion and the nerves by riding; the arms and hams by strong rubbing them daily.

d. The studious ought to have stated times for exercise, at least two or three hours a day; the one-half of this before dinner, the other before going to bed.

e. They should frequently shave, and frequently wash their feet.

f. Those who read or write much should learn to do it standing; otherwise it will impair their health.

g. The fewer clothes any one uses by day or night, the hardier he will be.

h. Exercise, first, should be always on an empty stomach; secondly, should never be continued to weariness; thirdly, after it, we should take to cool by degrees, otherwise we shall catch cold.

i. The flesh brush is a most useful exercise, especially to strengthen any part that is weak.

j. Cold bathing is of great advantage to health; it prevents abundance of diseases. It promotes perspiration, helps the circulation of the blood, and prevents the danger of catching cold. Tender persons should pour water upon the head before they go in, and walk swiftly.

To jump in with the head foremost is too great a shock to nature.

5. a. Costiveness cannot long consist with health; therefore care should be taken to remove it at the beginning, and when it is removed, to prevent its return by soft, cool, opening diet.

b. Obstructed perspirations (vulgarly called catching cold) is one great source of diseases. Whenever there appears the least sign of this, let it be removed by gentle sweats.

6. a. The passions have a greater influence upon health than most people are aware of.

   b. All violent and sudden passions dispose to, or actually throw people into acute diseases.

   c. Till the passion which caused the disease is calmed, medicine is applied in vain.

   d. The love of God, as it is the sovereign remedy of all miseries, so in particular it effectually prevents all the bodily disorders the passions introduce, by keeping the passions themselves within due bounds; and by the unspeakable joy and perfect calm serenity and tranquility it gives the mind, it becomes the most powerful of all the means of health and long life.

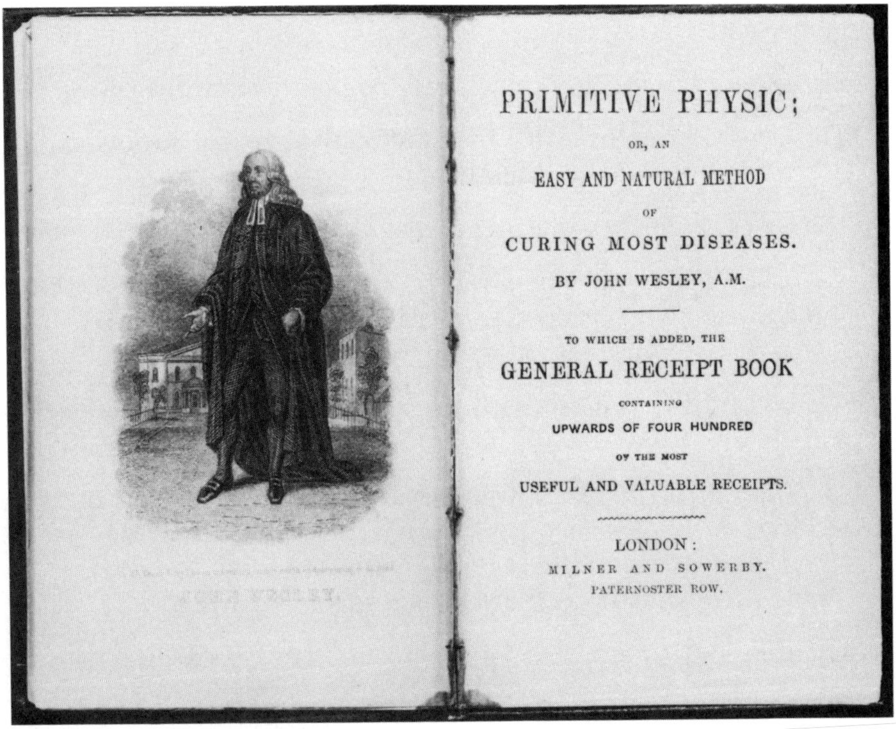
PRIMITIVE PHYSIC;

OR, AN

EASY AND NATURAL METHOD

OF

CURING MOST DISEASES.

BY JOHN WESLEY, A.M.

TO WHICH IS ADDED, THE

GENERAL RECEIPT BOOK

CONTAINING

UPWARDS OF FOUR HUNDRED

OF THE MOST

USEFUL AND VALUABLE RECEIPTS.

LONDON:

MILNER AND SOWERBY.

PATERNOSTER ROW.

Archives of the United Church of Canada

Pointers About Health

Rev. H. T. Crossley

The end of the 19th century was an era of religious and moral revival which included the growth of the temperance movement. All denominations encouraged and sponsored a variety of evangelical activities. One of the best known evangelistic teams during this period was that of Crossley-Hunter. The Rev. Dr. Hugh T. Crossley (1850-1934) and the Rev. John E. Hunter (1856-1919) came together in Ontario in 1884. It was claimed that, over the next 30 years of their joint ministry and revival meetings, more than 100,000 converts were made to Christianity.

While Crossley and Hunter were of the Methodist persuasion, their revival meetings in both large and small communities drew individuals of all denominations. The minutes of the June 1919 meeting of the Methodist Church, London Conference, noted the following:

> The scope of their work included every class from every walk in Canadian life. The writer saw in the great revival at Queen Street, Toronto, men fresh from prison soundly converted in the meetings. In one memorable meeting three drunkards were reclaimed, who became successful leaders. Among the better known converts were the late Sir John A. Macdonald, Premier of Canada, and Sir William Hearst, Premier of Ontario.

The Rev. H. T. Crossley published *Practical Talks on Important Themes (to young converts, older Christians and the unconverted)* (William Briggs, Toronto, 1895) which contained 31 addresses including, "Is Life Worth Living?", "Be a Consistent Christian," "The Parlor Dance," "The Cards," "The Weed" and "Pointers About Health." He believed that the moment of death is not pre-ordained by God. Rather, it is determined by one's regard or disregard for God's natural laws. If one observes these, one is assured of ample time to develop his or her intellectual and spiritual self. For, as Rev. Crossley concludes in his address on "Pointers About Health", selective excerpts from which are presented below, "We should seek to live on earth as long as possible, neither wearing or rusting out before our time."

We should make it part of our religion to look after our physical health. There are certain simple laws of health which, if all knew and practised, it would be well for the individual and the race.

1. Pure air - All persons should keep their bedroom windows open at night, summer and winter, and thus constantly sleep in fresh air, and so avoid breathing again and again their poisoned breath.

2. Suitable diet - Persons should avoid eating too much, too little, too fast, or too often.

   Drinking while eating is an unnecessary and injurious habit, which every one should avoid.

   There is a great deal of Christianity in good cooking and proper eating. Three meals a day, at set times, with about five hours between the meals, are as much as any person needs. We should eat to live and not live to eat.

   I have personally known men, and even ministers, that have died of stomach troubles; having been killed by poor cooking and indiscreet eating.

   Liquor and tobacco should be avoided. They are great causes of disease and death.

3. Exercise - Work is a primary law of health. Indolence makes people weak, sick, lack appetite and die prematurely, who, had they been energetic and industrious, would have been healthy, had a good appetite and lived for many years more.

4. "Cleanliness is next to godliness." Three-fourths of the earth's surface is water, hence, as it is so cheap and abundant, let us use plenty of it. Paul enjoins, "Cleanse yourself from all filthiness of the flesh."

   The pores of the skin should be kept open by bathing and perspiring. If a man's body were varnished all over, thus closing the pores or sewers, he would die in a short time.

   Will you permit me, in a couple of paragraphs, to express a few thoughts, not as an evangelist, but as a physician might address you.

   A great cause of disease and death in towns and cities is bad sewerage. Your body is a city; hence, if the sewers are clogged, the health will be greatly interfered with and life endangered. Costiveness is the clogging of the colon, or lower bowel, which is the main sewer of the body. This is a fruitful source of headaches, indigestion, dyspepsia, catarrh, jaundice, piles, liver and kidney troubles, sore eyes, skin eruptions and a host of other ills, physical, mental and moral. Bad sewerage of the body is abominable uncleanliness. Costiveness should be obviated, not by cathartic pills or purgative medicines—as the more of such are taken the more is required—but by diet, such as porridge, fruit at meals and at night, drinking water before retiring and after rising, and, when other means are necessary, by using an enema of from one pint to two quarts of pure water, about blood heat, retaining the water for a few minutes. Wisely employed, the enema will prove a great benefit to youths and adults. It should not be used, however, except when necessary.

5. Proper clothing - Wool should be worn next to the skin in winter and summer, by young and old. An Irishman, speaking of a woollen shirt, said, "Be it ever so wet and cold, it is always warm and dry."

   A suitable epitaph over many a grave would be, "Died from wearing thin-soled shoes and low-necked dresses."

   I shall not speak of corsets; suffice it to say that they prevent abdominal breathing, deform the body, lessen beauty, injure health, and prepare the way for unmentioned troubles. Many of the best and wisest families are abandoning corsets, while other people who laugh at and pity the Chinese for deforming their feet still adhere to cramping the waist, which is much worse.

6. Sleep is nature's benediction. Sleep all you can, but do not lounge in bed. The amount of sleep generally required by adults is from seven to nine hours. Every one, as far as possible, should have a regular time for retiring and rising, as we have for our meals.

7. Recreation is a good thing. According to political economy there are three departments in life: business, culture and recreation. "All work and no play makes Jack a dull boy." Every man and woman, as well as every boy and girl, should unstring the bow, so to speak, and every day take some pure and healthy recreation.

8. Medicine is sometimes necessary to help nature, but do not make a drugstore of yourself by continually swallowing medicine. "Do thyself no harm." Thank God for good physicians. Next to a minister, every physician, in order to be fully qualified for his important profession, should be a Christian, as was "Luke, the beloved physician."

9. A contented and peaceful mind may be possessed by everyone. Paul said, "Godliness with contentment is great gain," and affirmed, "I have learned, in whatever state I am, therewith to be content." Grace and resolution will develop the same experience and habit in each of us.

We should study, know and observe the laws of nature, for if these laws are transgressed the day of reckoning will come sooner or later. Being a Christian, or minister, sincere or ignorant, will not exempt any one.

If many who are now sickly, have no appetite, and are taking tonics and other medicines, would get their minds off themselves, go to work, exercise in open air, eat healthful food, keep good-natured and trust in God, they would soon be well.

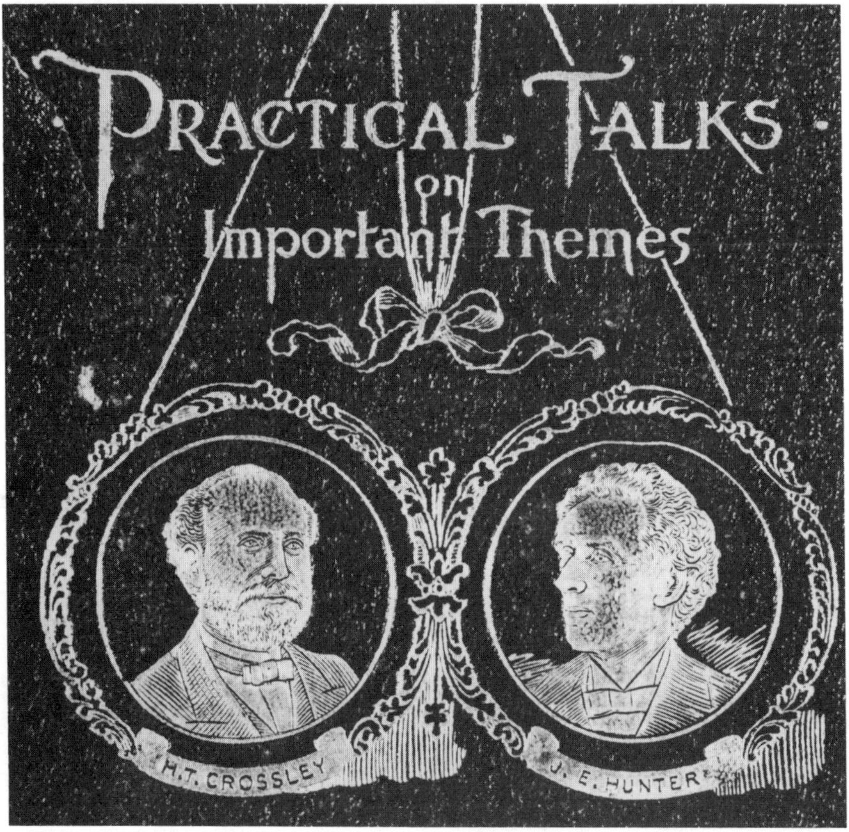

Advice For Good Health

Since the Ten Commandments were given to Moses on the Mount, we have been fascinated with self-improvement. If we only followed ten, easy steps, life's cup would overflow with milk and honey, and all would be bliss. The Victorians were no exception. In fact, they were positively obsessed with "do's and don'ts" and publications, like *The Household Guide*, frequently listed prescriptions for a better life.

True to its title, this book's main emphasis is on the treating and curing of ailments. However it only makes sense to refer briefly to some of the recommendations and advice of the time on how to avoid such illnesses in the first place. More often than not, there is an ironic correlation between the amount of advice available for preventing an ailment and the number of remedies proffered for curing that same ailment. Take, for example, colds, coughs, and sore throats. Advice abounds, yet obviously wasn't or couldn't be heeded—the number of remedies for treating cold-related illnesses far outweighs the amount of advice for preventing the same.

There is probably nothing new under the sun, or at least nothing which we have read or learned recently, that refutes the majority of the following advice. Personal responsibility, taken together with moderation and common sense, went a long way in the 19th century and there is no reason to believe that they are not as valid today.

Rules For The Preservation of Health

1. Adopt the plan of rising early, and never sit up late at night.
2. Wash the whole body every morning with cold water, by means of a large sponge, and rub it dry with a rough towel, or scrub the whole body for ten or fifteen minutes with flesh-brushes.
3. Drink water generally, and avoid excess of spirits, wine, and fermented liquors.
4. Sleep in a room which has free access to the open air, and is well ventilated.

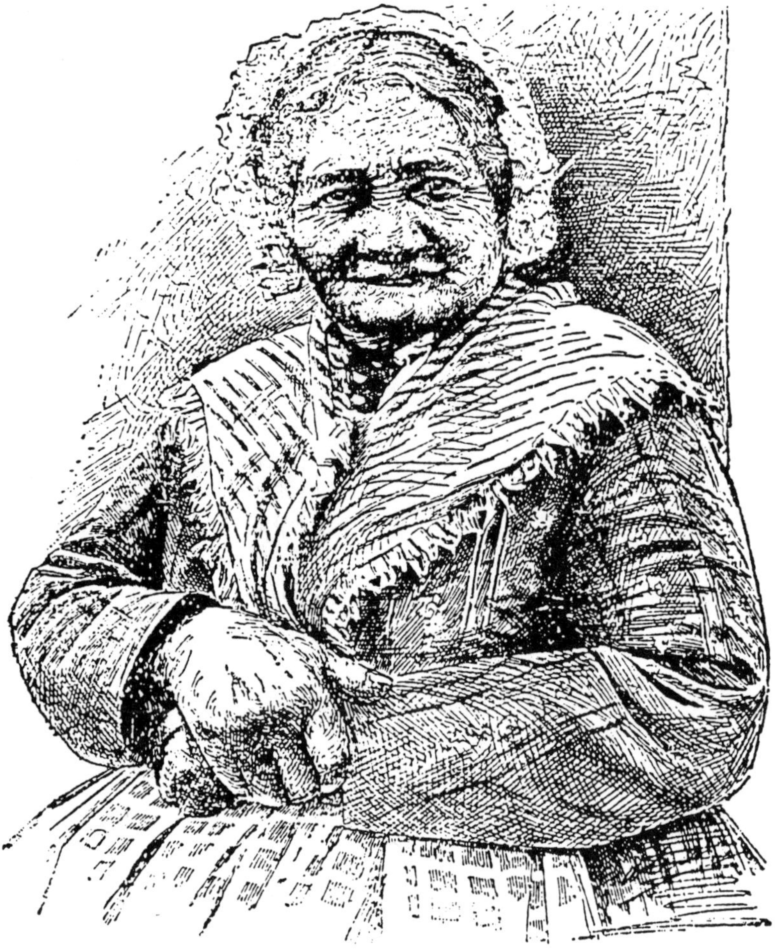

RIPE OLD AGE.

5. Keep the head cool by washing it with cold water when necessary, and abate feverish and inflammatory symptoms when they arise, by preserving stillness.

6. Symptoms of plethora and indigestion may be corrected by eating and drinking less per diem for a short time.

7. Never eat a hearty supper, especially of animal food; and drink wine, spirits, and beer only after dinner.

8. Exercise regularly adopted conduces to preserve health, and should always be taken by those who value so inestimable a blessing.

Mrs. Clarke's Cookery Book, Toronto, 1883

Life Lengthened - Sensible Rules For

Dr. Hall, in his excellent *Journal of Health*, gives the following sensible and suggestive rules:

1. Cultivate an equable temper; many have fallen dead in a fit of passion.
2. Eat regularly, not over thrice a day, and nothing between meals.
3. Go to bed at regular hours. Get up as soon as you wake of yourself, and do not sleep in the day-time—at least, not longer than ten minutes before dinner.
4. Work in moderation, and not as though you were doing it by the job.
5. Stop working before you are very much tired - before you are "fagged out."
6. Cultivate a generous and accommodating temper.
7. Never cross a bridge before you come to it; this will save you half the troubles of life. (In other words, "don't borrow trouble.")
8. Never eat when you are not hungry; nor drink when you are not thirsty.
9. Let your appetite always come uninvited.
10. Cool off in a place greatly warmer than the one in which you have been exercising. This simple rule would prevent incalculable sickness and save thousands of lives every year.
11. Never resist a call of nature, for a single moment.
12. Never allow yourself to be chilled through and through; it is this which destroys so many every year, in a few days' sickness, from pneumonia—called by some, lung fever—or inflammation of the lungs.
13. Whoever drinks no liquids at meals will add years of pleasurable existence to his life. Of cold or warm drinks, the cold ones are the most pernicious. Drinking at meals induces persons to eat more than they otherwise would, as any one can verify by experiment; and it is excess in eating which devastates the land with sickness, suffering and death.
14. After fifty years of age, if not a day labourer, and sedentary persons at forty, should eat but twice a day—in the morning, and about four in the afternoon; for every organ without adequate rest will "give out" prematurely.

15. Begin early to live under the benign influence of Christian religion, for it "has the promise of the life that now is and of that which is to come."

Dr. Chase's Third, Last and Complete Receipt Book, 1890, p. 168

❀❀❀

Practical Health Rules

1. It is no doubt a fact that health is at the command of most people. If people are sick, it is generally their fault, and not their misfortune. It is the violation of the laws of health that produces disease.

2. The average life in America would be about eighty years if proper care were taken of the mind and body; at present it is only thirty-four years.

3. To avert cold feet, wear two pairs of stockings, one pair of cotton or silk, the other of wool, and the natural heat of the feet will be preserved if they are kept clean.

4. Late hours and anxious pursuits exhaust the system, and produce disease and premature death. Therefore the hours of labour and hard study combined should be short.

5. Be moderate in eating and drinking; eat simple and plain food, avoid strong drink, tobacco, snuff, opium, and every excess, and your life will be lengthened many years.

6. A mild temper, and a serene and placid disposition will preserve health and lengthen life.

7. Never eat at irregular intervals. Regularity of meals is a necessity if dyspepsia and other forms of indigestion are to be avoided. Some persons are continually munching cakes, apples, nuts, candies, etc. This practice cannot be too severely condemned.

8. Never overload the stomach. Eating too much is about as bad as swallowing the food whole. The stomach is unable to digest the food, and it consequently ferments and produces disease.

9. Late suppers should always be avoided. Persons who indulge in hearty suppers never secure as sound sleep as those who eat lightly early in the evening.

10. Food should always be of good quality. Stale vegetables, which have lain in the market and withered for a long time, or fruit that is not perfect, is very injurious to the health.

11. One of the most essential things to health is a regular and vigorous system of bathing. Remember that "Cleanliness is next to Godliness."

The Household Guide, 1899, p. 73

❀❀❀

Ill Health - How Many People Bring It Upon Themselves

1. By eating too fast and too much.

2. By not chewing the food enough to make it fine, slushing it down with too much fluid, all through the meal.

3. By drinking spirits, or intoxicating drinks, too freely and too frequently.

4. By keeping late hours at night and sleeping it off in the forenoon.

5. By wearing too tight clothing, which prevents a free circulation of the blood.

6. By wearing too thin shoes and not protecting the feet from dampness and cold.

7. By neglecting to take sufficient exercise to keep the feet and hands warm.

8. By neglecting to wash and rub the body with a coarse towel, sufficiently to keep the pores of the skin open, for the escape of the effete, or worn out matter, of the system.

9. By changing the warm clothing of the day for light and inefficient, to attend evening parties.

10. By starving the stomach, as some do, to have enough to gratify the frivolous passion for dress.

11. By being constantly in a fret and worry, lest this or that shall not go as desired, or, in other words, borrowing trouble.

12. By eating and drinking at any or all hours of the day or night, instead of eating at regular hours and in only moderate quantities—nine-tenths of the people eat twice as much as is necessary to sustain life and health.

Dr. Chase's Third, Last and Complete Receipt Book, 1890, p. 82

Health Rules For Winter ~ Colds & Inflammation

1. Never lean with the back upon anything that is cold.
2. Never begin a journey until the breakfast has been eaten.
3. Never take warm drinks and then immediately go out in the cold air.
4. Keep the back, especially between the shoulders, well covered, also the chest well protected.
5. In sleeping in a cold room, establish the habit of breathing through the nose, and never with the mouth open.
6. Never go to bed with cold or damp feet; always toast them by a fire 10 or 15 minutes before going to bed.
7. Never omit weekly bathing, for, unless the skin is in active condition, the cold will close the pores and favour congestion or other diseases.
8. After exercise of any kind, never ride in an open carriage or near the window of a car for a moment; it is dangerous to health and even to life.
9. When hoarse, speak as little as possible until it is recovered from, else the voice may be permanently lost or difficulties of the throat be produced.
10. Warm the back by a fire, and never continue keeping the back exposed to heat after it has become comfortably warm; to do otherwise is debilitating.
11. When going from a warm atmosphere into a colder one, keep the mouth closed so that the air may be warmed by its passage through the nose ere it reaches the lungs.
12. Never stand still in cold weather, especially after having taken a slight degree of exercise; and always avoid standing on ice or snow, or where the person is exposed to cold wind; in short, keep your feet warm, your head cool, and your mouth shut and you will seldom "catch cold."
13. To the foregoing rules from "Common Sense" allow the Old Doctor to make a "baker's dozen" of them, by saying that the most fruitful seed from which colds, and often consumption arise, is the pernicious habit of young people loitering at the gate. Never do it.

Dr. Chase's Third, Last and Complete Receipt Book, 1890, pp. 123-124

Practical Rules For Bathing

1. Bathe at least once a week all over, thoroughly. No one can preserve his health by neglecting personal cleanliness. Remember, "Cleanliness is akin to Godliness."

2. Only mild soap should be used in bathing the body.

3. Wipe quickly and dry the body thoroughly with a moderately coarse towel. Rub the skin vigourously.

4. Many people have contracted severe and fatal diseases by neglecting to take proper care of the body after bathing.

5. If you get a good reaction by thoroughly rubbing in a mild temperature, the effect is always good.

6. Never go into a cold room, or allow cold air to enter the room until you are dressed.

7. Bathing in cold rooms and in cold water is positively injurious, unless the person possesses a very strong and vigourous constitution, and then there is great danger of laying the foundation of some serious disease.

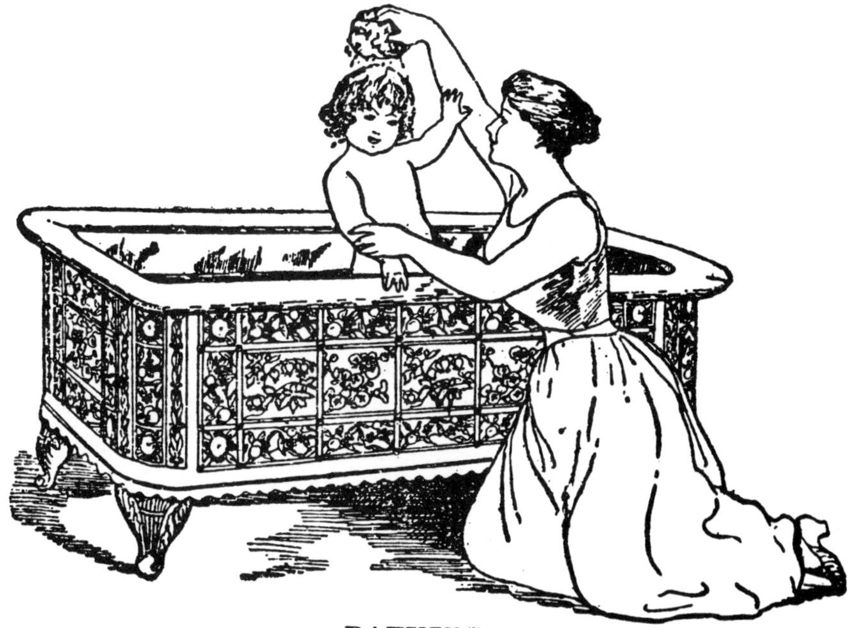

BATHING.

8. Never bathe when the body or mind is much exhausted. It is liable to check the healthful circulation.
9. Never bathe within two hours after eating. It injures digestion.
10. A good time for bathing is just before retiring. The morning hour is a good time also, if a warm room and warm water can be secured.
11. Never bathe a fresh wound or broken skin with cold water; the wound absorbs water, and causes swelling and irritation.
12. A person not robust should be very careful in bathing; great care should be exercised to avoid any chilling effects.

The Household Guide, 1899, p. 68

❀❀❀

How To Keep A Baby Well

1. The mother's milk is the natural food, and nothing can fully take its place.
2. The infant's stomach does not readily accommodate itself to changes in diet; therefore, regularity in quality, quantity and temperature is extremely necessary.
3. Not until a child is a year old should it be allowed any food except that of milk, and possibly a little cracker or bread, thoroughly soaked and softened.
4. Meat should never be given to very young children. The best artificial food is cream, reduced and sweetened with sugar and milk. No rule can be given for its reduction. Observation and experience must teach that, because every child's stomach is governed by a rule of its own.
5. A child can be safely weaned at one year of age, and sometimes less. It depends entirely upon the season, and upon the health of the child.
6. A child should never be weaned during the warm weather, in June, July or August.
7. When a child is weaned it may be given, in connection with the milk diet, some such nourishment as broth, gruel, egg, or some prepared food.
8. A child should never be allowed to come to the table until two years of age.

9. A child should never eat much starchy food until four years old.

10. A child should have all the water it desires to drink, but it is decidedly the best to boil the water first, and allow it to cool. All the impurities and disease germs are thereby destroyed. This one thing alone will add greatly to the health and vigour of the child.

11. Where there is a tendency to bowel disorder, a little gum arabic, rice, or barley may be boiled with the drinking water.

12. If the child uses a bottle it should be kept absolutely clean. It is best to have two or three bottles, so that one will always be perfectly clean and fresh.

13. The nipple should be of black or pure rubber, and not of the white or vulcanized rubber. It should fit over the top of the bottle; no tubes should ever be used. It is impossible to keep them clean.

14. When the rubber becomes coated, a little coarse salt will clean it.

15. Babies should be fed at regular times. They should also be put to sleep at regular hours. Regularity is one of the best safeguards to health.

16. Milk for babies and children should be from healthy cows. Milk from different cows varies. Some authorities insist that it is better for a child to have milk from the same cow, while others prefer mixed milk from a herd, as less liable to changes.

17. Many of the prepared foods advertised for children are of little benefit. A few may be good, but what is good for one child may not be for another. So it must be simply a matter of experiment if any of the advertised foods are used.

18. It is a physiological fact that an infant is always healthier and better to sleep alone. It gets better air and is not liable to suffocation.

19. A healthy child should never be fed oftener than once in two hours, gradually lengthening the time as it grows older; at 4 months 3 1/2 or 4 hours. At 5 months a healthy child will be better if given nothing in the night.

20. Give an infant a little water several times a day.

21. For colds, coughs, croup, etc., use goose oil externally and give a teaspoonful at bed-time.

The Household Guide, 1899, pp. 221-22

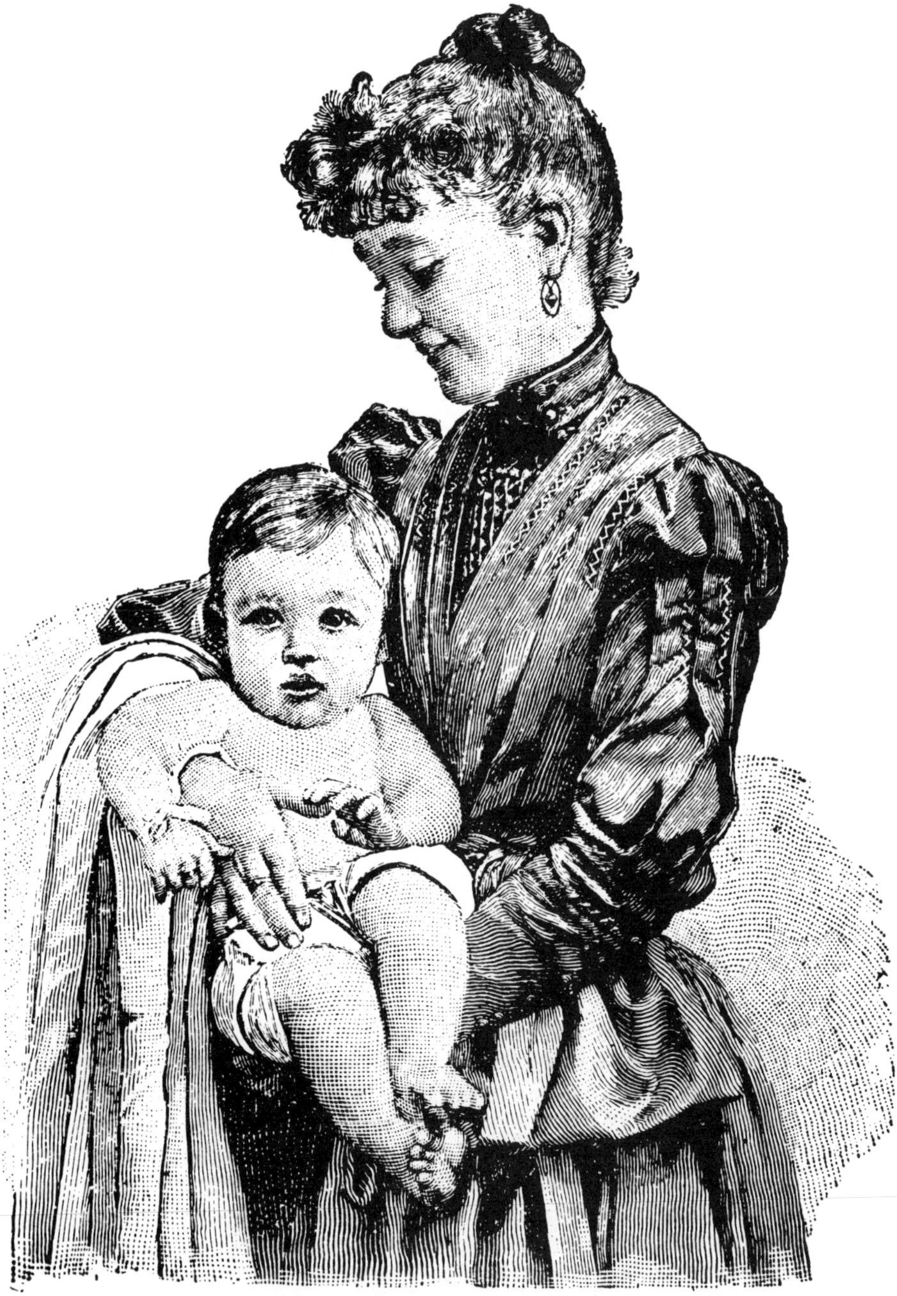

A WELL CARED-FOR BABY.

Aphorisms

- The windows opened more would keep doctors from the door.
- The best physicians are Dr. Diet, Dr. Quiet, and Dr. Merryman.
- Excess calls in the doctor.
- Eat not to dullness—drink not to elevation.
- Disease is the punishment of neglect.
- Keep the blood pure and spare the leech.
- Loose habits lead to tight bandages.
- Bottles of brandy are followed by bottles of physic.
- Be temperate in all things.
- Keep the head cool and the feet warm.
- Better pay the cook than the doctor.
- Health is the reward of cleanliness.
- Moderation is a great safeguard.
- The healthiest feast costs the least.
- A good suggestion is often invaluable.
- There is no balm for every wound.
- Observation is the best teacher.
- Pure water is better than foul wine.
- Guard well the steps of the useful.
- Prevention is better than cure.
- The quiet mind enjoys the sweetest rest.
- Where reason rules appetite obeys.
- Eating and drinking shouldn't keep us from thinking.
- We seldom repent of having eaten too little.
- Life's but a means unto an end.

Enquire Within Upon Everything,
65th Edition, London, Houlston & Sons, 1882

Folk Medicine

The primary focus of this book is on self-help remedies from the 19th century—remedies which were published in household guides, receipt books and newspaper and magazine articles. That being said, the fact can not be ignored that many people turned to the remedies found in folklore when searching for a way to cure an ailment. These folk remedies were not recorded on paper, but rather passed by word of mouth from neighbour to neighbour and from generation to generation. The study of Canadian folklore, of which folk medicine is a part, has appropriately developed into an important, although an often unknown, part of our cultural history. The following examples of folk medicine are noted, not only as a contrast to self-help remedies, but also to emphasize the range of minority medical practices which were prevalent in 19th century Canada.

Folk medicine is structured on a belief system of mysticism, magic, or religion transferred through cultural communities for hundreds of years. In the context of our "modern" perspective, these often can only be "rationalized" for their placebo effect. At the same time we are beginning to recognize or understand again that good or bad health can be affected by one's beliefs and by one's frame of mind.

The following examples of folk medicine, while perhaps bemusing to read, should not be dismissed as mere curiosities; rather they should be noted because of their widespread usage and perceived credibility in their time. Treatments based on folk medicine as well as self-help remedies could, and likely were, used at the same time for the same ailments. Indeed it is not possible to identify with any certainty which of these approaches might have been tried first. However, as the 19th century progressed, with a more settled and educated community, folk medicine began to play a much less important role in communities where it had once been strong.

Waterloo County, Ontario

Bee Stings

If you can succeed in killing the bee that stings you the wound will not mortify.

Colic

If before breakfast on Easter morning you suck a raw egg that was laid on Good Friday, it will keep you from getting the colic the rest of the year (Amish).

Consumption

A tea made from the feces of a black horse was once prescribed as a cure for pulmonary trouble.

Cure For Bad Temper

Pass the child head first through the left leg of its father's trousers.

Dog Bite

Take some of the hair of the dog that bit you and place them in the wound.

For The Eyes

Wear earrings for sore eyes.

Take the blood of a bat and bathe your eyes with it and you will be able to see as well in the dark as you can in the daytime.

Cures For Fits

Give the blood of a black hen as a drink to the patient.

Some to cure a child thus afflicted took it into the woods, placed it with its back against a tree, and bored a hole into the tree above the child's head. They then cut off some of the child's hair and stuffed it into the hole, which they closed with the wooden plug. It was believed that as the child grew up above the hole the disease disappeared.

A Pennsylvania German told me that, if a person who was subject to fits found a horseshoe with the nails still in the holes, he was to remove them and have them made into rings. These, he said, would have a salutary effect if worn by the afflicted person.

Freckles

Dew rubbed on the face before sunrise on any morning during the month of May will remove freckles and give one a beautiful complexion.

Cure For Goitre

To cure goitre or thick neck wind a black ribbon around the neck three times and then put the ribbon into a coffin with a corpse, but do it secretly.

Rub the hand of a corpse on the goitre.

Rheumatism Cure

Carry a horse-chestnut in the pocket.

The skin of a white weasel worn about the person is regarded as a preventative.

Cure For Rupture

Take the hand of a corpse and press the thumb on the rupture and it will be cured.

Cure For Side-stitch

Spit on a pebble and throw it over your shoulder, and then walk away without looking back at it.

Another cure is to overturn a stone and spit into the cavity in the soil caused by its removal and then replace the stone.

For Sore Throat

Take the sock off your left foot, turn it inside out, and wear it around your neck. It is said the cure will be more effectual if the sock is red.

Cure For Sore Umbilicus

Get a hen's egg from your neighbour and hold it on the child's umbilicus until the egg is warm, then bury it where the rain will not fall upon it, and as it decays the sore will heal. This must be done before sunrise, and during the performance you are not to speak to anyone.

For A Sprain

If you find a bone, run it on the sprained hand or foot, and then throw it over your shoulder and do not look back.

Sties

Throw a pail of swill over your head without wetting yourself.

Toothache Cures

Cut off a bunch of your hair and place it with a corpse in a coffin. This must be done secretly.

If a child chews a bread crust that has been gnawed by a mouse it will never be subject to toothache.

A bone from a pig's skull, called hern-zahn (i.e., "brain-tooth"), is carried in the pocket as a preventive. It is also worn suspended around a child's neck to assist in teething.

A splinter from a tree that had been struck by lightning if used as a toothpick will prevent toothache.

Cure For Warts

Rub a copper coin on the wart and present it to some person who will thereupon get it.

Get into a house and steal a dishcloth and bury it under a stone; as the cloth rots the wart will also disappear.

Take a potato and cut in two and then rub one of the pieces on the wart. Take this and wrap it in a piece of paper and place it on the sidewalk or other place much frequented by the public. Whoever opens the package will get the wart.

If you have more than one wart on your hand get some person to count them and he will get them.

Whooping Cough

Let the child eat a piece of bread from the hands of a woman whose maiden name was the same as her husband's surname.

Another cure is to take the hair of a person who has never seen his or her father alive and put it on the child's breast.

Birthmarks

It is claimed that a birthmark will assume the colour of a strawberry at the times this fruit is ripe; but as soon as the strawberry season is over, it resumes its normal colour.

Death and Burial

When a wild bird enters an occupied house one of the occupants will soon die.

If the clock strikes 6 or 12 while the head of the house asks the blessing it is a sign of a death.

A Charm For Toothache

Before sunrise or after sunset go to a spring on a neighbour's farm and take three mouthfuls of water (not with a cup but with the mouth) and spit them on the ground, at the same time invoking the Trinity three times. This is to be done for 3 nights in succession, and you are not to speak to anyone while doing it.

> *Selected from W. J. Wintemberg,* Folk-Lore of Waterloo County, *Ontario, National Museum of Canada, Bulletin No. 116, Ottawa, 1950. See also , W.J. Wintemberg, "German-Canadian Folk-Lore",* Ontario History, *Vol. 3 (1901), pp. 86-96.*

❀❀❀

Folklore From Ontario

Bleeding

The seventh son of the seventh son can stop haemorrhages, as can also the seventh son.

To stop nose-bleed, place a key or a coin on the back of the neck.

A black ribbon tied about the throat prevents nose-bleed.

Goitre

For goitre, wear a string of beads about the neck.

The seventh son can cause goitre to disappear by rubbing.

Rub the neck three times with a green frog, which is then thrown away. The goitre will disappear. Another remedy consists in touching the goitre with a live frog. The animal is then buried head downwards in the ground. As the frog decays, the goitre will disappear.

Warts

Take some gravel from the lake shore, rub it on the warts, then wrap it up and throw it away.

Take a string and tie as many knots in it as you have warts, then throw it away. As the string rots, the warts will disappear.

Scratch the warts with a match, and then make a scratch on the stove-pipe. When the scratch disappears, so do the warts.

Steal a pod of green peas at midnight in silence and secrecy, shell it with eyes shut, and rub each pea on a different wart, then wrap them in paper and bury.

Take a hair from a gray horse, wind it around the wart, and hide it under a stone.

Headache

To throw the combings of one's hair out of doors causes headaches when the sun shines upon it.

Never throw combings from your hair out of doors, for the birds may take them to build their nests, and you will have a headache.

Don't rock an empty cradle; it will make baby's head ache.

Teeth

To secure good, sound teeth, as the milk-teeth were extracted each girl swallowed them. The son, who refused to swallow his teeth, was the only member of the family who had an unsound tooth in his head.

When a child loses a tooth, he should cast it over the left shoulder, or burn it, so that its successor will come in straight.

Whooping Cough

If a child has the whooping cough in the spring before the leaves are out, the cough will leave when the leaves open; if during the summer, the cough will leave when the leaves go.

Stye

A stye may be cured by rubbing with a wedding-ring, or even with a gold ring (according to some).

Hiccough

For hiccough take three drops of water in the name of the Father, Son and Holy Ghost.

Selected from F. W. Waugh, "Canadian Folklore from Ontario"
Journal of American Folk-Lore, *Vol. 31, 1918, No. 119, 120.*

Les Remèdes d'Autrefois
Champlain County, Quebec

Boils

Eat lead shot in odd numbers.

Palpitation of the Heart

Cut out a heart in red cloth and wear it on underclothes next to the heart.

Corns

Squash a frog between the big toe and the second.

Rheumatism

Go into the forest, cut a notch in a tree and say: "Rheumatism, I'm leaving you; when I come by again I'll pick you up."

Consumption

Drink the urine of black cow.

Convulsions in Children

Take their shirt off, turn it inside out and burn it.

Cramps

When you go to bed, put your shoes upside down.

Tetter

Put a wedding ring or a nun's ring around it.

Toothache

Carry the head of a fish in your pocket.

Cut your finger nails on Monday.

Wear a walnut on a string around your neck.

Sore Throat

Take off the sock from your left foot, and apply the bottom of it to your throat.

Haemorrhoids

Carry a piece of sealing wax in your pocket.

Carry a horse chestnut.

Apply the suet of a black ram.

Incontinence of Urine In Children

Make them eat roast mouse.

Make them eat mouse droppings.

Leg Trouble (aches)

A foot bath in "running water" on St. Jean de Baptiste Day helps aches and pains in legs for the whole year.

Jaundice

Eat an uneven number of lice.

Eat lice on your bread and butter.

Whitlow

Apply the excrement of a black cow.

Nose Bleed

Say five Paters and at the same time turn something upside down.

Sweating

To stop your hands from sweating, choke a mole in your left hand.

Warts

When you see a shooting star, say "Go away wart," and the wart disappears.

Put as many peas into a bag as there are warts. Throw the bag behind you onto the road over your shoulder without looking at it. Whoever picks up the bag will get your warts.

Eye & Earache

Rub with "thunder wood," that is to say wood which has been struck by lightning.

Selections from a translation of "Les Remèdes d'autrefois," collected by E. Z. Massicotte in Champlain County, Quebec (1890-1895) in Journal of American Folk-Lore, *Vol. 32, pp. 176-178. See also William R. Riddell, "Some old Canadian folk medicine,"* The Canadian Lancet and Practitioner, *Aug. 1934, pp. 41-44.*

Lunenburg County, Nova Scotia

Asthma

Take three locks of hair from the crown of a child's head, spit on it three times and put it in a piece of paper. Bore a hole in the door casing the height of the child's head and plug the paper in the hole. As the child grows above the hole the asthma will leave him.

Garden Lots, Mahone Bay and Blandford

Cramps

For cramps in the legs, when you go to bed at night turn your shoes upside down with the heels up.

Mahone Bay

Drink

To cure a man of drink take an eel and put in rum, but don't leave the eel in long enough to die. Then give the rum to the person to drink, but don't tell him about the eel. If he drinks it he will never touch rum again.

Lunenburg

Fits

If a child has fits we would split an oak tree and put the child in. If the oak grew the child would get better, but if not, the child would die.

Blockhouse

Nose Bleeding

If a child has nose bleeds bore a hole in the door. Take a lock of hair from the top of his head and parings from his fingers and toe nails and put in a paper. Place in the hole in the door, which is at his height. As he grows above the hole the nose bleeding will stop.

North River

Warts

Take three beans and rub the warts an uneven number of times, the same as the number of warts you have. Bury the beans and as they rot the warts will go away.

Rose Bay

Selected from Helen Creighton, Folklore of Lunenburg County, *Nova Scotia, National Museum of Canada, Bulletin No. 117, Ottawa, 1950*

Thanks For The Memories

The many remedies which I found in books, newspapers, and other publications from the late 1800s and early 1900s provided confirmation of what I had perceived to be the case—that the concerns and conversations about one's health and the many methods to improve it have had a central place in the Canadian social fabric, ranked closely with our discussions about the weather and politics.

With this thought in mind, I wrote in 1993 to community newspapers and chapters of Women's Institutes across the country hoping to get firsthand recollections of home remedies which had been remembered and saved from the past. The response was overwhelming and leaves me in the regretful position of being able to publish a mere sampling of the letters received. I thank all of the contributors for their letters, advice, and anecdotes.

The section which follows contains some of these letters. Home remedies and cures in the self-help tradition still remain, although in a diminishing way, in personal recollections, oral history, and family tradition. Most of the letters were written by women in their seventies, eighties, and nineties who passed on family recipes as well as family remembrances. In an important sense, this should not have been unexpected as women have been by practice, if not by necessity, the traditional caregivers in most families and communities. A most appreciated and unexpected component of the letters was the offering of their mementos—offers to send worn copies of family cookbooks or photocopies of pages which they thought I might find relevant; personal anecdotes of how their families dealt with all sorts of diseases and ailments; and lists of sources which they remembered from childhood.

Common threads ran through the letters. Writers from Nova Scotia told of similar cures for warts and earaches as did the contributors from Saskatchewan. People from across the country referred to books such as *The Household Guide* and various editions of Dr. Chase's "receipt books" and took the time to explain how these works came to be in their possession.

My requests for information struck a chord of memory containing a mixture of down-to-earth practicality and nostalgia.

"My recollection of the various home remedies that my mom used is vivid though I cannot for the life of me remember if they actually brought relief. But, I suppose that they must have. We just were unable to afford conventional medicines."

Marjorie Batchelder, Thunder Bay, Ont.

❀❀❀

"Yesterday as I read your ad in the P.E.I. Journal, you won't believe the memories it brought back from years gone by but, before I go any further, I must ask you to excuse my writing as I am French and not very good at writing in English. Back to my stay when I was a child, I come from a family of ten and my parents were very poor. They could not afford a doctor everytime one of us was sick so they made their own medicine and believe me it worked every time. I will tell you a few remedies that I can remember."

Helen Blanchard, Summerside, P.E.I.

❀❀❀

"I am sending you some examples of home remedies handed down from my mother and mother-in-law and their mothers before them. I am from a family of ten children and, as you must be aware of, in those days there was not any money to waste, nor any emergency wards, so they took care of us at home and when all else failed the family doctor was summoned. I hope some of these will be of use to you, and I would like to say I still use them on my family when necessary."

Olive Dewar, Vankleek Hill, Ont.

❀❀❀

The tone and detail of these letters were uniformly positive, whether from a young mother in rural Alberta, two senior citizen sisters receiving home care in Bruce County, Ontario, or members of the Women's Institute from Bay Roberts, Newfoundland. What do the following responses indicate? The answer to this question is that the home remedies and cures which were in common use one hundred years ago have not yet disappeared from living memory—although unfortunately they likely soon will.

The heading for this section was inspired by one of the many letter-writers, Ethel Poth of Maple Grove Lodge, Goderich, Ontario, who noted, *"Success is limited in having these elderly people remember home remedies for me, all of us being in our eighties and nineties. Our forgetteries are better than our memories."*

Arthritis

I remember, when we would visit, as a child and young teenager picking waist-high thistles for Ma (paternal grandmother) to boil up for her "tea." She would make "tea" in the summer when the thistle bloomed [had a pink-purple "flower" (tuft) on it]. Then we would put it in her freezer so she'd have it all winter (reheated, of course), for her arthritis.

Donna Latramouille, Yellowknife, N.W.T.

Bronchial Coughs

Store remedy for coughs was Electric Oil which I remember tasted good but according to our mother was not good and was too costly. If my father had not got into the closest town in the fall and brought back "White Lightning," i.e. Homebrew for Medicinal purposes usually in a long necked beer bottle with cork, this was given to us by a teaspoonful. However, failing this we got a teaspoonful of coal oil and sugar. It was effective but hard to swallow.

Pamela Menard, Riverton, Man.

Constipation

My mother also used this method for constipation. You had to drink more than a half a cup of sauerkraut juice.

Mrs. M. E. McLeod, Gimli, Man.

Head Lice

When I was about 12 years old we had a house guest that left us with head lice. Living on a farm we had not a lot of money. My dad soaked our hair and heads with kerosene oil, then wrapped them with a steaming hot towel. Next came the fine tooth comb. Ten days later if one nit were found we were in for the same torture.

Helen MacLean, Borden, P.E.I.

Fever

For a high fever she would put fish (herring) on our forehead (it worked). The fever would be so high it would cook the fish.

Helen Blanchard, Summerside, P.E.I.

Bad Eyes

In case we would have bad eyes when we grew up they made sure we ate carrots every day, and it worked and is still working.

Mrs. Tilmon J. Arsenault, Wellington, P.E.I.

Rusty Nail Wound

I remember well when I was about 7 years old of stepping on a rusty nail and this nail stuck in the centre of my foot. Grandma pulled the nail out and applied a poultice made of cow's milk and chunk of bread. This was put on a wool rag as hot as I could stand it and tied on my foot. When it cooled down it was again heated and applied. After several applications Grandma looked at my foot and said it would now heal and it did.

Mildred Merrill, Bayfield, Ont.

Insect Bites

For insect bites, take a broad leaf plantain leaf or leaves, wash to remove any soil etc., pour boiling water over the leaves to sterilize, place over the bite or injury and cover with a bandage to hold in place. You may have to do this several times.

Mary Culbert, Ripley, Ont.

Wakefulness Cure By Lemon Juice

The wakefulness that comes from drinking too strong tea or coffee can be conquered by swallowing a dash of fresh lemon juice from quartered lemon, placed in readiness on the bedside table, and taken at the time you discover that sleep will not come.

Annie Volk, Humboldt, Sask.

High Fever

When I was a tiny baby (1906), I developed a very high fever. The doctor had my mother pack me in ice! In 1915, for a high fever, *that* doctor had me wrapped in a steaming hot wool blanket (wrung out of very hot water). Since I am still alive, you can see that the opposites both worked.

Ethel Poth, Goderich, Ont.

Stings, Ingrown Toe Nails, Boils, Etc.

This is most effective in drawing infections, i.e., stings, ingrown toe nails, boils, etc. Take a small amount of brown soap (laundry) such as "fels naptha;" work with a spoon or knife until soft. Work in a small amount of brown sugar, a little moisture may be added to make it pliable. The original moisture was spittle. Apply directly to the area, and cover with a soft cloth or band aid. This is a family remedy, brought from the Isle of Tiree, Scotland in the 1850s.

Sara Speiran, Kincardine, Ont.

Influenza

This was used in the influenza epidemic of 1918. Give the patient a hot bath; then with arms held close to their sides, wrap them snugly in a wool blanket. This was done by rolling the patient and blanket over and over until the full length of the blanket was used. Leave over night and in the morning the sweat soaked blanket was removed and the patient kept warm for a few days.

Camilla Cline, Coronation, Alta.

Colds And Flu

In early spring and fall—use lots of cinnamon—this helps to ward off colds and flu. Cinnamon toast, rather than making a mixture to spread. Use cinnamon as pure as you can, then sprinkle with sugar or pack of sugar substitute to taste.

Marjorie Marshall, Palmerston, Ont.

Poison Ivy

To "cure" poison ivy my mother placed a copper penny in a cup and half-filled the cup with vinegar. She let this sit over night. The penny turned partly green. She dabbed this vinegar on my brother's poison ivy blisters. He "danced" on the kitchen floor and walked away "cured." This cup sat on our kitchen window sill for weeks until the poison ivy season was over.

Bertha Tiessen, Brantford, Ont.

Bronchial Congestion & Fever

Once in my practice as family physician, I was called to the home of a six-month-old child, where the problem was bronchial congestion and fever. Before I could examine the baby, I had to remove several slices of white Italian bread soaked in red wine, from her chest. Unfortunately, I did not enquire (as I should have) about how this bread/wine poultice was intended to work for the baby's healing—but I did not discourage the mother from applying it again to her child!

Lois F. Hazen, M.D., L. W. Pubnico, N.S.

Earache

I am an old girl (80 this July) and so these remedies were used on me. My grandparents and parents didn't believe in bothering a Doctor for minor ailments, unless their home cures didn't work. When I had earache my dad blew tobacco smoke in my ear, or I had the inside core of an onion stuck in my ear.

Rosamond Allen, Yarmouth, N.S.

Cough Medicine

1 cup fancy molasses; 1/2 cup white sugar; 2 tbsp. vinegar; 1 onion (cut fine); 2 tsp. ginger. Boil strain and bottle. Take a teaspoon whenever needed. This heals the lungs.

My mother used this recipe to raise four children, alone, only had a Dr. Book to go by. This is her own recipe though. She once had a very sick young man to care for and used this cough medicine. They claim she saved his life.

Lucy Phinney, Trenton, Ont.

Earache

One of my memories shared by my sisters was, if we as youngsters had an earache, our Dad who smoked cigarettes would take a bit of tobacco from his pouch "chew it" and put it in our ear. He would put us on his knee and pat us and we now wonder if it was not the fact of being held and comforted that did the trick or would there be a bit of heat from the tobacco? As we got older I remember camphorated oil, warmed, put on a bit of cotton ball tucked into the ear. This would be in the 1920s and 30s.

Mrs. M. Gibson, Paris, Ont.

Coughs

For coughs our own cough syrup was made. An onion was sliced into a handleless cup to about the halfway mark (I'm not sure why a handleless cup but that was what Mother always used). Then the cup was filled with brown sugar and allowed to sit overnight. A spoonful of the resulting light brown liquid soothed the throat and stopped the cough.

Elaine LaMarche, Elrose, Sask.

Stomach Cramp

The Lang family emigrated from Odessa, Russia in the early 1900's to Devils Lake, North Dakota. In 1904 the family trekked to the Scott, Saskatchewan area and in 1906 my husband's parents married and homesteaded in the Revenue area. The old homestead is still standing. One family remedy was dill seed, brewed into a tea for stomach cramps.

Ann E. Lang, N. Battleford, Sask.

Chest Cold/Cough

Mom raised some geese in the summer and, come autumn, these sassy birds would end up in the freezer, ready to be cooked. Christmas would arrive as always and we would have a lovely roast goose dinner with the trimmings. As you probably know, the goose's flesh is, or tends to be, "oily" and there would be "grease" at the bottom of the pan. This "grease" was saved and stored in a clean container, either in the fridge or the freezer.

Whenever someone had a heavy chest cold and a harsh cough, Mom would take the goose grease, after it had softened some (at room temperature) and rub some on the cold sufferer's upper chest and throat. The area was warmly covered and the cold sufferer was sent to bed. The cold would be "loosened" by morning (usually) making life easier for the victim.

Jan Graham, LeRoy, Sask.

Gall Stones

A number of years ago Edith Hood told me a story about how she was cured of a gall stone problem. Edith was in her forties at the time of her troubles. The time would have been the early 1930s. One of her neighbours in Muskoka told her a way to be free of gall bladder problems.

1) Fast for 2 days.

2) Mix 2 cups of olive oil and the juice of a grapefruit.

3) Drink this mixture and wait for the result.

Edith passed her stones and wasn't troubled again by her gall bladder. She lived a long life of a hundred or so years.

Sheila C. McCaskill, Huntsville, Ont.

Earache Home Remedy

For earaches, my mother would heat about 2-3 cups of table salt in a frying pan until it was hot to the touch. She would then take a piece of flannel material (flannel because it was warmer and softer to the touch—about 14" x 14") and lay it on a flat surface and pour the salt onto the piece of flannel. She would then gather up all the sides and with a piece of string, tie it up so that it resembled a bag. She would then make us lie down and she would put the bag of heated salt under our ear and we would lie on it until the salt began getting cool. We would sometimes have to put another cloth on top of the bag because it was too hot but it usually worked and has worked for my family.

Mary J. MacVicar, Leamington, Ont.

Sore Throat

When I was a little girl (1931) and had a sore throat my mother found a wool sock in the laundry basket (preferably stiff from perspiring) and pressed that to my throat and wrapped it around my neck. I don't know if the smell or the wool cleared up my sore throat in record time!

Margaret Toews, Leamington, Ont.

Good Advice

When our children grew up and got married with families of their own (we had 5 children—3 girls and 2 boys), I would offer suggestions to them for cradle cap, etc. Well I soon learned not to suggest anything to them. Everything today must be by the book when raising children. Funny, I don't think that babies have changed over the last few centuries. The doctor knows everything, even if it costs money to cure.

Pat Fortune, Guelph, Ont.

Arthritis/Rheumatism

For arthritis and rheumatism take 1 tablespoon pure Cod Liver Oil; 3 tablespoons strained orange juice.

Keep in the fridge in small jars and shake well before taking. Take 4 hours after last meal of the day. Take for 3 months for best results. The above is for *one* dose.

Anna Allison, Douglastown, N.B.

Blood Poisoning

I thought I would send along a few things I remember my parents and myself used. I am 83 so have seen a bit of the past. For blood poisoning take an old wool underwear and put on a bed of hot coals from the cook stove in a bucket. Put the affected part in the smoke.

Alice (Doll) Ahlgrim, Didsbury, Alta.

Upset Stomach/Dysentery

Every year in the 30's and 40's we drove 15 miles north from our farm to do some blueberry picking. This was tubs full and cream can fulls. These were processed in quart jars. It was used as a dessert, but it also was used as a healer of an upset stomach or when we suffered with dysentery. Mother would fetch the jars and give us the juice to drink.

Valerie Bleakney, Saskatoon, Sask.

Balm of Gilead Salve

My grandmother used to make a salve which was extremely useful. As kids we called it "Bam - a - giled." The recipe was as follows:

4 lbs mutton tallow

3 oz. elder bark

4 oz. bamagiled buds

3 oz. tobacco

Stew these in tallow; then strain and add 3 oz. of powdered rosin and 3 oz. beeswax. Heat till dissolved. Put in tin boxes while warm. Get the buds while they are sticky.

This was a wonderful healing salve if applied lightly. When my father was a youngster, he cut his arm quite severely. Since getting to the Doctor 8 miles away presented a problem, my Grandmother dressed the wound with her salve. Later, when the Doctor saw the arm, he told my Grandmother that it had healed better than it would have if it had been stitched.

Carol A. Robbins, High River, Alta.

Sore Throat

Take 4 or 5 little potatoes, roast on coals until tender. Put in an old stocking and crush it on the floor with your foot. Hold it steaming hot to the throat three or four times until trouble disappears. After this is taken off, grease throat and chest well with camphorated oil.

Carolyn Taylor, Dartmouth, N.S.

Croup

Drops of coal oil on sugar for croup.

My brother says if we had all the coal oil in one jug that we ate on sugar we could keep a lamp lit for a long time. As I recall we burped coal oil for the next two days after the dosage.

Mrs. Glenn Wiley, Clinton, Ont.

Cold And Sore Throat

Put a dirty sock around your throat, for a cold or a sore throat.

Esther Gibbs, Frankville, Ont.

Constipation

My great-uncle Tommy would sit on a pail of hot water (steaming). It was supposed to help relieve constipation. He would do this in the winter out behind the wood shed. It would look funny with the steam coming out all around him.

Betty Gemmill, Clayton, Ont.

Healing Wounds

Last but not least was the dreaded of all whey bath. This stuff stank to high heaven and I would only use it if I had to or in desperation. Whey had some type of medicinal healing properties, which I still don't understand, it was used for cleaning and healing wounds. I tried it once when a teenager to clean up acne but couldn't stand the smell. It was also used for ulcers, yes, some folks drank it.

Joney Benting, Hay River, N.W.T.

Croup

In Yarmouth where I lived as a small child an Indian told my mother (maybe 1907-08) about a cure for croup which my brother had. Take equal part of bear's grease and salt—spread on a flannel rag and put on the chest. It works now even if you use lard to mix with the salt.

Elizabeth A. Lavers, Chester, N.S.

Blood Poisoning

A little boy got blood poison in his arm in winter-time. Lettuce saved him, it was very hard to find lettuce in winter, none even in Renfrew. The butcher shop man sent someone to Ottawa and got some there. It had to be pounded up to get the juice out of it. However it worked.

Pearl Easton, Williamsburg, Ont.

Cough

When I was 12 years old I drank a bottle of ice cold soft drink on a very hot day. It was on July 12th, at a school picnic. I started coughing and coughed for about 4 weeks. Mother tried everything she could think of and nothing helped. One day a salesman came. He was a Hebrew and asked mother why on a hot day I am wearing a towel wrapped around my neck. She told him my problem. He said you give her—1 beaten egg, 1/2 cup warm milk, 1/4 tsp. sugar and a couple of drops vanilla. Mix that and give her 3 times a day to drink. I stopped coughing before school started. I still use this remedy when I get a bad cough and it helps.

Mary Dobko, Yorkton, Sask.

Sick of School

For "sick of school," go back to bed and mother will give you a dose of castor oil, tried and true and the surest cure I ever did see.

Olive Dewar, Vankleek Hill, Ont.

Bowed Legs

I had 2 brothers and when quite young were very bow legged. My dad took the eldest into a bone specialist in Winnipeg and he wanted to break the legs and re-set—my dad said, "In no way will the legs be broken."

Shortly afterwards my dad read an article on the same subject—when the ground is warm in the spring, put a bow-legged child barefooted on the green grass. This worked for both boys.

Mrs. D. Matthewson, Stonewall, Man.

Bruises

A pet dog's tongue soothed lots of bruises.

Dora Rutherford, Oro Twp and Orillia, Ont.

Colicky Babies

I was told by an elderly German lady to get fennel tea for my colicky babies. I made the tea in a pot exactly the same way as if making regular tea for myself. After it was cooled, I put approximately 4 oz. and 1 teaspoon of white sugar in a nursing bottle (sugar helps to prevent choking and soften stool). It is given whenever required.

Barbara Alcorn, Hillsborough, N.B.

Measles

Around about 1890 my mother tells the story that she and her sister had measles. If the rash did not come out they were given a home remedy. My mother said that as they were going to bed she heard their mother (my grandmother) say to their father that if the rash did not come out in the morning she would give them "The Remedy"—*IT WAS SHEEP MANURE!*

I do not know if she mixed it with anything but she tells or I should say told us that in the morning her rash came out but her sister's did not and she got the Sheep "S."

Through the years mother would tell us the story and my aunt would get really annoyed at her for telling us about it. The harder we laughed the angrier she got.

Verna Munroe, Campbellton, N.B.

Diarrhoea And Vomiting

This is my most valuable recipe, which I credit with saving my daughter's life. At age approximately 3 months, my daughter came down with a severe bout of diarrhoea and vomiting which lasted about a week. She had not slept in 3 or 4 days and was so weak she could not even cry any more. I was scared stiff. I took her to the local hospital emergency—and they were full up at the hospital—and said to just watch her.

Then I remembered reading an article in a farm magazine—about using cow colostrum to save calves with scours. The first dose I gave her: a couple of teaspoons diluted about half and half with water. The diarrhoea eased, and she slept for the first time in days. When she woke I gave her more, this time diluted 4 to 1 with water, and added a dash of corn syrup. The diarrhoea stopped and I carried on this treatment for 3 days, before returning to other food. She was completely cured.

Therese Siemers, St. Paul, Alta.

Fractured Jaw

My father was hit by a train while crossing the track (naturally) and as I was told they used cow flaps as a poultice for a presumably fractured jaw.

Marguerite K. Vontobel, Carleton Place, Ont.

Cuts

I was a toddler in the summer of 1906 and of course wanting to help my mother pick choke cherries to make that scrumptious jelly we grew up on. They tell me I was standing on a box to reach the cherries and fell off onto a tin my mother was using. The edge was very sharp and I had a bad cut on my nose. Mother didn't panic or rush me to a doctor. She first applied ordinary white flour to stop the bleeding. I still have a scar but no doubt would have even if I had had stitches.

Jean Holmes, Carleton Place, Ont.

For Worms

Whether children had any symptoms of having worms it seemed that they needed treatment. Our speciality was one drop of turpentine on a half teaspoon of white sugar. I think we were allowed to take a sip of water afterwards. Three evenings in succession then skip three days. Continued for a series of nine days. Atrocious!!

Ruby Greer, Stanstead, Que.

Kidney and Bladder Infection

Pumpkin seeds that had been washed, dried then boiled, about 1/2 cup seed to 1 cup of water sweetened. We used this for kidney or bladder infection and also if we had trouble urinating, especially new-born babies; if they couldn't urinate were given a weak pumpkin seed tea sweetened with brown sugar. This I had given to my sister when I was only 16 years old. It seemed to work.

Minnie Priebe, Chesley, Ont.

Bee Sting

When picking raspberries with my mother, if I got stung with a bee, she would say "Spit on the spot and rub some dry dirt in it to make a paste—let it dry on." It helped.

Marian Mainprize, St. Mary's, Ont.

Gangrene

Fresh raw pig skin can eliminate gangrene from badly infected sores, cuts, any broken skin. Place the fat side onto skin taping it tightly to skin and placing bandage over top of that. Check every eight to ten hours for replacement of pig skin. No meat must be on pig skin patch, just a thin layer of fat attached to the outer skin. Must be fresh, uncooked, unsmoked, uncured pig skin only. What the pig skin does is basically suck all infection out of the area.

Jenny Callsen, Newbrook, Alta.

Anaemia

A pale person, suspected of being anaemic, was given rhubarb jam for breakfast, rhubarb pie for lunch, and rhubarb sauce for supper as rhubarb was high in iron. Eating rhubarb raw, straight from the garden is highly recommended.

Gladys Doherty, Westlock, Alta.

Mustard Plaster For Severe Bronchitis

When a mustard plaster was required for severe bronchitis, it was a mixture of bread flour, powdered edible mustard (Keen's mustard in the 1930s) and perhaps a little baking soda (I don't remember the quantities of each of the ingredients).

This was mixed into a paste by adding and mixing in gradually a limited amount of warm water until the mixture was semisolid or creamy. This was spread on brown paper and applied with the mustard mixture directly in contact with the skin of the chest. After approximately ten minutes the paper was removed with most of the flour-mustard mixture still adhering to the paper. The residue on the skin of the chest was washed off with lukewarm water and some vaseline jelly (failing that, some melted grease from the skin of a cooked goose, called of course, "goose grease") was applied gently to the reddened human skin of the chest.

Ralph Haldenby, Guelph, Ont.

Codfish Oil

Quite often we had to take raw codfish oil, and what a putrid taste. My mother would go down to Pictou, N.S., where the fishermen had cod in barrels and salvage the raw fish oil that settled on the top, she would skim this off. These barrels would be sitting in the hot sun, so you can just imagine the smell.

John R. Fraser, Gagetown, N.B.

Oil Of Smoke For Ringworm Or Skin Blemishes

For ringworm or skin blemishes, wipe the blade of an axe—place in a safe position. Burn brown paper on the blade—drops of sweat will form—rub on infected skin.

Margaret Newson, Barrie, Ont.

High Fever

Just as a matter of interest, I am listing a few home remedies given to me by my mother who is 82 and, apparently, were used by her grandmother. The interesting aspect is they all seemed to work!

For high fever apply a piece of very fat pork to the soles of the feet and wrap.

Dorothy M. James, Trenton, Ont.

Dog Bite

Make a poultice of laundry soap and saliva and place on a dog bite for twenty-four hours.

Jean Harvey, Gull Lake, Sask.

Spring Tonic

It was my mother's firm belief that in spring we needed to have our blood purified, I guess to eliminate winter's blah or as a spring tonic. Anyway, we were dosed with a mixture of sulphur and molasses daily for a week or so. Whether it purified our blood I'll never know but it certainly cleared the bowels and the resulting gas did nothing to family closeness until the period of purifying came to an end.

Irene Toverud, Viking, Alta.

Rash

One fellow told me he had such a rash on his face and an old lady told him to wash his face in his urine and he told me look at my face, it's all cured and I did it only once. It sounds odd but you never know.

Johanne Chegil, Kamsach, Sask.

Corn

My father had a corn on the sole of his foot and did this and has had no more problems. First you get a pan of water as hot as you can stand and a pan of very cold water. Soak your foot in the hot water for 5 minutes, then quickly dip it in the cold water for 1 second. Do this several times for an hour. Then while your foot is hot dip it in a pan of coal oil. You are to do this everyday for several days (Dad said he only did it once).

Carol Perrin, Carrot River, Sask.

Diarrhoea

It is called White Man's Door Mat for diarrhoea and it worked good. You gather it out in the yard and bring it in and pour water on it and boil it a bit and use the gruel to drink for the diarrhoea. Not much of white man's door mat is around now as most places are sowed to grass. I can remember it around the house on the farm.

Mildred Beaudoin, Maymont, Sask.

Rusty Nail

If someone stepped on a nail—the dreaded "rusty nail"—one of us was sent to pick "raw wool" from the barb wire fence. Sheep would often squeeze under the bottom wire and thus leave tufts of wool on the barbs. (Washed wool could not be used.) This wool was set on fire, to smoulder in the dustpan, while the patient held his foot over the thick, yellow smoke for at least 30 minutes—always out on the back porch—the smell was awful. This remedy must have worked, for no one unfortunate enough to step on a nail ever developed blood poison and the pain wasn't felt again.

Edra M. Campbell, Stony Plain, Alta.

Gathering

When I was a child I had frequent infections in my fingers, around the finger nail. The finger became badly swollen—the infection was known as a "gathering." My mother removed the crusts from a slice of bread (preferably home-made), put it in a small dish and poured boiling water over it. The water was quickly squeezed out, the damp, hot bread put on a piece of cloth, and wrapped around the finger over the infection. Left on until it was cold, this bread poultice reduced the fever and eventually killed the infection.

Mrs. G. M. Astley, Irma, Alta.

Prairie Itch or Seven-Year Itch

The Prairie Itch or Seven-Year Itch (scabies) was caused by a mite that got under the skin. Take a bath every day, then rub down with iodine and goose grease, sulphur and lime, or powdered sulphur and lard.

Dianne Taubert, Hussar, Alta.

Arthritis

When I was 59 years old I had arthritis in my back. I thought it was a pinched nerve, so I went to the doctor. X-rays showed it was arthritis. The doctor said: "There is no cure for arthritis, you will just have to learn to live with it. At your age you can consider yourself lucky you haven't had it sooner." He gave me a sample of pain killers. I went home and threw them in the garbage and decided I would find a cure. It took a while but I finally made a tea from the leaves of Canada thistle. It not only cured me but everyone that has tried it has had very good results. I am 75 years old now and have no signs of arthritis.

Ruby M. Sterr, Glendon, Alta.

Toothache

I grew up in a rural farm area twenty-five miles to the nearest dentist. This was before the days of medicare and money was not plentiful. So when we got a toothache we tried all sorts of remedies to ease the pain. Whole cloves packed into the cavity of the tooth helped. Or, sometimes a few drops of liniment from an eye dropper into the tooth helped for a few days but invariably we would end up at the local doctor and he would pull the tooth out in his office.

Laura Williams, Copetown Women's Institute, Dundas, Ont.

Snow Blindness

For snow blindness, place onions on your eyes.

Adeline Legrow, Bauline, Nfld.

How To Preserve Children

Take: 1 large grassy field; 1/2 doz. children; 2 or 3 small dogs; a pinch of brook and some small pebbles. Mix the children and dogs well together and put them in the field stirring constantly. Pour the brook over the pebbles, sprinkle the field with flowers, spread over all a deep blue sky, and bake in a hot sun. When thoroughly browned, remove and set to cool in a bath tub.

Maureen Margetts, Williams Lake, B.C.

A Grandmother's Cold and Flu Cure

Garlic—in foods, flavourings or essence, it works. Even the germs can't stand it! It was first discovered during the "Spanish Flu" epidemic following World War I. The previously scorned immigrants from Central and Eastern Europe did not get ill, why? Garlic.

Ethel Cuts, St. Albert Women's Institute, St. Albert, Alta.

Cod-Liver Oil

A health practice which was administered universally in the 1930s was the distribution of cod-liver oil. School-aged children were given their dose by their teachers every morning at school. For those who had children who were unable to attend school, parents would bring their own bottle from home to the local store and fill it up (at no charge) with cod-liver oil from a large wooden barrel. Everyone was expected to take their daily dosage. Cod-liver oil was also credited with reducing the pain and inflammation of arthritis and rheumatism. Also, a variation to the bread poultice was to make a paste from mussel shells which had been dried in the oven until brittle, powdered and mixed with hot water as you would a bread poultice.

William and Una Smith, Trinity Bay, Nfld.

Epilogue

Now that one has arrived at the conclusion, we should perhaps ask ourselves where this has led us. Canada in the 19th century was a young country undergoing significant social and economic change in the transition from pioneer, to established rural, to emerging industrial urban communities. Hundreds of thousands of emigrants from Europe had brought with them their own traditions of self-help medicine, which they of necessity or by choice came to depend upon in their new environment.

It was a time of pre-modern evidence-based medicine when many individuals and families were required to deal with their own ailments. Of course, we have no way of knowing in detail the extent of the use of these particular self-help remedies. Indeed, at a given moment in one home, a variety of different ailments were likely to be treated with a combination of folk medicine, self-help treatments (using readily available natural ingredients), or patent medicines. The cure was all that was really important, and which remedy or treatment had done the trick was often only to be surmised about later.

James Burke, in commenting on monks of the Middle Ages who spent their days recopying ancient manuscripts, notes that "all they knew was old." In a significant sense our perspective on the current practice of medicine is that "all we know is new." Nevertheless, we are beginning to see a growing appreciation of the importance of a return to more natural and less intrusive medical treatments and an awareness of the importance of personal responsibility for one's own health. The past indeed does have something to teach us.

Glossary

Anodyne - A medicine which will allay pain.

Aperient - A gentle laxative or purgative.

Astringent - A drug which seems to cause contraction of the tissues. Used to diminish discharges, such as ulcers of the skin, etc.

Balm - Aromatic and fragrant medicine, usually an ointment.

Catarrh - Flow of mucus from the nose or other parts of the body.

Cathartic - A drug that increases the action of the bowels.

Decoctions - Made by adding a pint and a half of water to an ounce of the plant or herb, boiling down to one pint, and straining while hot.

Diuretic - A remedy which increases the quantity of urine excreted.

Emetic - Medicine which produces vomiting.

Expectorant - Medicine that produces free discharges from the lungs or throat.

Extracts - Made by adding a small amount of alcohol to the bruised leaves, or other parts of the plant. The juice is thus extracted, and is placed in a warm place to evaporate until it becomes as thick as honey.

Flux - Diarrhoea, or other excessive discharges.

Fomentations - Bags of herbs wrung out of hot herb teas and applied to the affected parts.

Itch - Scabies. A catching eruption of the skin, accompanied by severe itching.

Nostrum - A quack preparation, usually of the patent order.

Powders - Made from finely broken up or pulverized barks and herbs.

Receipt - Archaic form of the word recipe.

Teas or Infusions - Made by pouring boiling water on the plant or bark and allowing it to steep for a short time until the water cools, after which the liquid is strained. Sometimes cold water is used.

Tinctures - Solutions of the medical properties of herbs in alcohol or in mixtures of alcohol and water.

Tonic - A remedy which increases the strength of the individual either by supplying some element which his system lacks, such as iron, or by improving the condition of his stomach so that this organ is better able to digest and absorb the nutritious elements of the food.

Vermifuges - Medicines to expel worms.

Approximate Measures

- A teacup contains four fluid ounces, or one gill.
- A wineglass contains two fluid ounces.
- A tablespoon contains one-half fluid ounce.
- A teaspoon contains one-eighth fluid ounce, or one dram.
- Sixteen large tablespoonfuls make half a pint.
- Eight large tablespoonfuls make one gill.
- A scruple is an apothecary's weight unit of 20 grains.

HOFFMAN, WEGENAST & COMP'Y,

KING ST. EAST, WATERLOO, ONT.

MANUFACTURERS OF

Household Furniture!

WHOLESALE and RETAIL.

—o—

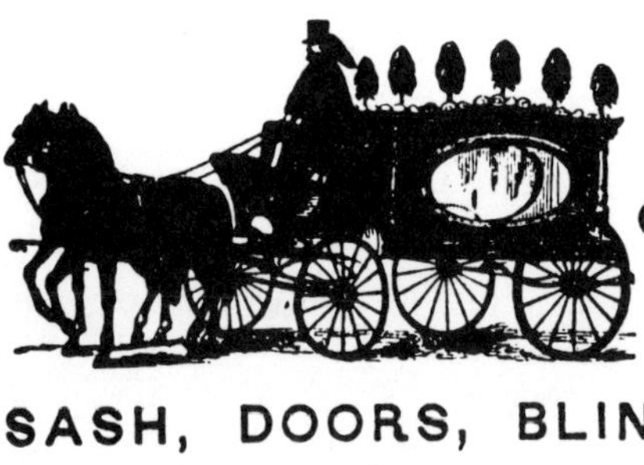

UNDERTAKING.

A FULL SUPPLY OF

Coffins, Caskets, Shrouds, and Good HEARSE

always on hand.

SASH, DOORS, BLINDS AND MOULDINGS.

—o—

☞ PLANING and MATCHING done to order. A large stock of LUMBER, LATH, and SHINGLES constantly on hand. Buildings of all kinds **erected in any style** required, and on reasonable terms.

County of Waterloo Gazetteer and Directory for 1877-8, Toronto, 1878.

Acknowledgements

Let me begin by acknowledging and thanking the archivists and librarians who not only have provided professional access to their holdings, but also have dealt in a friendly way with a stranger: Ellen Morrison and Darlene Wiltsie, University of Guelph, Guelph, Ont.; Lindsay Moir, Glenbow Museum, Calgary, Alta.; Margaret Mahone, Osborne Collection, Toronto Public Libraries; Dan Zelenyj, City of Vaughan Archives, Maple, Ont.; Ian Mason, United Church Archives, Victoria University, Toronto, Ont.

In addition, the following individuals, both previous friends and those I have met along the way, have helped me in a myriad of ways, not only by providing information, but also in the important sense that their interest in this book has served as an encouragement to see it through to its completion. I thank them all: Mr. and Mrs. Paul Baker, R.R. #2, Maple, Ont.; Gary Berssenbrugge, Ottawa, Ont.; Ian Bowering, Cornwall, Ont.; Don Boyes, London, Ont.; Vicki Busby, Napanee, Ont.; J. T. H. Connor, Hanna Institute for the History of Medicine, Toronto, Ont.; Mary Evans, Woodstock, Ont.; Alan Foster, MTRCA, City of Vaughan, Ont.; John R. Fraser, Gagetown, N.B.; Susan Grafi, Kleinburg, Ont.; Lorna and Al Jackson, Woodbridge, Ont.; Joan Lyons, Matapedia, Que.; John McCamus, Toronto, Ont.; Glen and Mary Norcliffe, Maple, Ont.; Brian Osborne, Kingston, Ont.; Norm Perry, Kincardine, Ont.; Janine Roelens-Grant, Federated Women's Institutes of Ontario, Guelph, Ont.; Katharine Schmidt, Guelph, Ont.; John Spanhouse, Mississauga, Ont.; Jack Warwick, Toronto, Ont.; Mrs. Alma Watson, R.R. #4, Brussels, Ont.; Debbie Thompson Wilson, Guelph, Ont.; Bill and Gail Wolfe, R.R. #1, Dobbinton, Ont.; Elaine Yates, R.R. #3, Tottenham, Ont.

Finally, let me note and thank the many individuals who wrote to me in response to my request for information on self-help remedies which they and their families have used. I hope that they will find in this book a reasonable presentation of their interest in this aspect of Canada's social history: Sadie Adam, St. Albert Women's Inst., St. Albert, Alta.; Alice Ahlgim, Didsbury, Alta.; Barbara Alcorn, Hillsborough, Alta.; Rosamond Allen, Yarmouth, N.S.; Marion Allen, Dalhousie, N.B.; Anna Allison, Douglastown, N.B.; M. Anguish, Brantford, Ont.; Mrs. Tilmon J. Arsenault, Wellington, P.E.I.; Emily Arthur, Grenfell, Sask.; Mrs. G. M. Astley, Irma Women's Inst., Irma, Alta.; Marjorie I. Batchelder, Thunder Bay, Ont.; Ernest & Mildred Beaudoin, Maymont, Sask.; Joney Benting, Hay River, N.W.T.; Betty Bethune, Waterdown, Ont.; Clara Black,

Campbellville, Ont.; Helen Blanchard, Summerside, P.E.I.; Valerie Bleakney, Saskatoon, Sask.; Edna & May Boyle, Holyrood, Ont.; Lyla Brocklebank, Orangeville, Ont.; Janet M. Brown, Simpson Women's Inst., Simpson, Sask.; Lillian Byer, Stouffville, Ont.; Jenny H. Callsen, Newbrook, Alta.; Edra M. Campbell, Stony Plain, Alta.; Cora Carlton, Melfort, Sask.; Roberta Chabot, McIrvine Women's Inst., Fort Francis, Ont.; Johanne Chegil, Kamsach, Sask.; Wilf H. Clark, Spencerville, Ont.; Camilla Cline, Coronation, Alta.; Alice Crandall, Elgin Women's Inst., Elgin, N.B.; Mary Culbert, Ripley, Ont.; Annie Danyluk, Canora, Sask.; Marie H. Darris, Kings Co., N.S.; Olive Dewar, Vankleek Hill, Ont.; Marilyn Dickie, Calgary, Alta.; Patricia Dix, Cambridge Stn., N.S.; Mary Dobko, Yorkton, Sask.; Gladys A. Doherty, Westlock, Alta.; Pearl Easton, Williamsburg, Ont.; Margaret Eddy, Brantford, Ont.; Doreen Empey, Iroquois, Ont.; Margaret W. Ferguson, Cobourg, Ont.; Marie Flegel, Nipawin, Sask.; Allan Forsyth, Tottenham, Ont.; Pat Fortune, Guelph, Ont.; Georgina Frair, Picton, Ont.; John R. Fraser, Gagetown, N.B.; Betty Gemmill, Clayton, Ont.; Esther Gibbs, Frankville, Ont.; Mrs. M. Gibson, Paris, Ont.; Sylvia Goeres, Canmore, Alta.; Jan Graham, LeRoy, Sask.; Lois J. Grant, Calgary, Alta.; Ruby Greer, Stanstead, Que.; Ralph Haldenby, Guelph, Ont.; Ms. M. E. Halley, Annapolis Royal, N.S.; Eileen Hamilton, Wroxeter, Ont.; Jean Harvey, Gull Lake, Sask.; Gloria M. Hastings, Amherst, N.S.; Dr. Lois F. Hazen, Pubnico, N.S.; Jean Holmes, Carleton Place, Ont.; Arthur Homer, Campbellton, N.B.; Evelyn Howden, Caledonia, Ont.; Jean A. Hume, Guelph, Ont.; Jane Hunter, Amherst, N.S.; Lyn Isaac, Camp Morton, Man.; Dorothy M. James, Trenton, Ont.; Vivienne Jarvie, Burnaby, B.C.; Margaret Jerome, Burnaby, B.C.; Mrs. C. King, Milford, Ont.; Ann E. Lang, North Battleford, Sask.; Donna Latramouille, Yellowknife, N.W.T.; Elizabeth A. Lavers, Chester, N.S.; Ann Leighton-Kyle, Vernon, Ont.; Grace Levy, Mahone Bay, N.S.; Hanna Lewis, Calgary, Alta.; Kathy Lindseth, Strome, Alta.; Eva Linklater, Burnham Women's Inst., Swift Current, Sask.; Carol Lowerison, Salisbury, N.B.; Mrs. Elden Lowry, Kincardine, Ont.; Helen Maclean, Borden, P.E.I.; Gladys Macleod, Roblin, Man.; Mary J. MacVicar, Leamington, Ont.; Marian Mainprize, St. Mary's, Ont.; Carrie Malott, Morpeth, Ont.; Elaine La Marche, Elrose, Sask.; Maureen Margetts, Williams Lake, B.C.; Marjorie Marshall, Palmerston, Ont.; Mrs. D. Matthewson, Stonewall, Man.; Bev G. McAlister, Dutton, Ont.; Sheila C. McCaskill, Huntsville, Ont.; L. Violet McLellan, Welwyn, Sask.; M. E. McLeod, Gimli, Man.; Pamela Menard, Riverton, Man.; Mildred Merrill, Bayfield, Ont.; Verna Munroe, Campbellton, Ont.; Margaret Newson, Barrie, Ont.; Jo Ann Nickerson, Kingston, N.S.; Anne Paine, Brantford, Ont.; Jean Patterson, Brooke Women's Inst., Alvintson, Ont.; Mrs. F. Pel, Burnaby, B.C.; Gwen Pemberton, Bayfield, Ont.; Carol Perrin, Carrot River, Sask.; Lucy Phinney, Trenton, Ont.; Alma Pinch, Leamington, Ont.; Ethel Poth, Goderich, Ont.; Minnie Priebe, Chesley, Ont.; Mrs. Carl Reid, Orangeville, Ont.; Beth Richardson, Annapolis County, N.S.; Carol Anne Robbins, High River, Alta.; Ruth Large, Baldonnel Women's Inst., Baldonnel, B.C.; Helen Seymour, Bay Roberts Women's Inst., Bay Roberts, Nfld.; Therese Siemers, St. Paul, Alta.; William & Una Smith, Trinity Bay, Nfld.; Jessie Smith, Arnprior, Ont.; Sara Speiran, Kincardine, Ont.; Ruth Steedman, Brantford, Ont.; Helen Steinburg, Cardinal, Ont.; Ruby M. Sterr, Glendon, Alta.; Frances Strain, Success Women's Inst., Success, Sask.; Dianne Taubert, Hussar, Alta.; Carolyn Taylor, Dartmouth, N.S.; Mary Taylor, Winchester, Ont.; Kay J. Thomas, Burnaby, B.C.; Bertha Tiessen, Brantford, Ont.; Margaret Toews, Leamington, Ont.; Irene Toverud, Viking, Alta.; Dorothy M. Turnbull, Whitehorse, Yukon; Joyce Turvey, Eastend, Sask.; Katharine H. Unger, Cremona, Alta.; Mary Urness, Ft. MacLeod, Alta.; Marguerite K. Vontobel, Carleton Place, Ont.; Russell Wallace, Halifax, N.S.; Mrs. Jim Watson, Chatham, Ont.; Alma Watson, Brussels, Ont.; Helen Weaver, St. Vincent Women's Inst., Meaford, Ont.; Mrs. Glenn Wiley, Clinton, Ont.; Laura Williams, Copetown Women's Inst., Dundas, Ont.

Helpful Guide For The Reader

The self-help remedies noted in this book are mainly contained in the section entitled, Good For What Ails You. The following partial index notes where specific topics are located in that section. In addition, a large range of specific remedies are found elsewhere in the book particularly in the section, Thanks For The Memories.

Endnotes

Preface

1. James Thomas Hamilton Connor, "Minority Medicine in Ontario, 1795-1903: A Study of Medical Pluralism and Its Decline")Ph.D. theses, University of Waterloo, 1989). This excellent work provides a clear and detailed overview of all aspects of minority medicine during this period.

Primitive Physic ~ John Wesley

1. *Collier's Encyclopedia,* vol. 19 (New York: P. F. Collier and Son, 1956): 426.

2. John Wesley, *Primitive Physic; or an Easy and Natural Method of Curing Most Diseases* (London: Milner and Sowerby, [1780?]): xiv-xvi. Held by United Church of Canada/Victoria University Archives, Toronto.

3. George Dock, "The Primitive Physic of Rev. John Wesley, "*The Journal of the American Medical Association,* 54 (1915): 629-638.

4. Eunice B. Bardell, "Primitive Physic: John Wesley's Receipts," *Pharmacy in History,* 21 (1979): 111-121.

5. John Wesley, *Primitive Remedies* (Santa Barbara, CA: Woodbridge Press, 1975).

John Crossley - Practical Talks

1. John Webster Grant, *A Profusion of Spires: Religion in Nineteenth Century Ontario* (Toronto: University of Toronto Press, 1988): 182.

2. *Christian Guardian* (June 18, 1919): 16.

3. *The Observer* (October 15, 1965): 24-26.

Folk Medicine

1. Edith Fowke, *Folklore of Canada* (Toronto: McClelland and Stewart, 1976).

2. Edith Fowke and Carole H. Carpenter, eds., *Explorations in Canadian Folklore* (Toronto: McClelland and Stewart, 1985).

3. Peter Morley and Roy Wallis, eds., *Culture and Curing—Anthropological Perspectives on Traditional Medical Beliefs and Practices* (Pittsburgh, PA: University of Pittsburgh Press, 1979).

4. Jennifer J. Connor, "Folklore in Anglo-American Medical Journals 1845-1897, " *Canadian Folklore Canadien,* 7 (1985).

Bibliography

Baker Papers, City of Vaughan Archives. Maple, Ontario.

Barnum, H. L. *Family Receipts: or Practical Guide for the Husbandman and Housewife*. Cincinnati, Ohio: A. B. Roff, 1831.

Bull, William Perkins. *From Medicine Man to Medical Man: A Record of a Century and a Half of Progress in Health and Sanitation as Exemplified by Developments in Peel*, Toronto, 1934.

Busby, Vicki Jean. "Doctors Can't Cure It: Traditional Medical Practices in Nineteenth Century Upper Canada: Survival Strategies in a Developing Society, 1783-1920." M.A. thesis, Queen's University, Kingston, 1993.

Canniff, William. *The Medical Profession in Upper Canada, 1793-1850.* Toronto: W. Briggs, *1894.*

Caplan, Ron, ed. *Down North, The Book of Cape Breton's Magazine*, Toronto: Doubleday Canada , 1980.

Chase, A. W. *Dr. Chase's New Receipt Book or Information for Everybody*. Toronto: Rose Publishing Co., n.d.

Chase, A. W. *Dr. Chase's Third, Last and Complete Receipt Book and Household Physician or Practical Knowledge for the People.* Memorial Edition. Detroit and Windsor: F. B. Dickerson, 1890.

Dr. A.W. Chase's Calendar—Almanac, Toronto and Buffalo: Dr. A. W. Chase Medicine Co., 1914.

Mrs. Clarke's Cookery Book comprising a collection of about fourteen hundred Practical, Useful and Unique Receipts. Toronto: The Grip Printing and Publishing Co., 1883. CIHM 01114.

The Common Sense Recipe Book Containing All The Latest Recipes On Cooking With Economy: And Also Very Valuable Medicinal Recipes. Montreal: John Lovell and Son, 1895.

Connor, James Thomas Hamilton. "Minority medicine in Ontario, 1795-1903: A Study of Medical Pluralism and Its Decline." Ph.D. thesis, University of Waterloo, 1989.

Dictionary of Canadian Biography, Toronto: University of Toronto Press, 1966.

A Directory of Medical Archives in Ontario. Compiled by Margaret Dunn. Edited by Mary Baldwin. Toronto: The Hannah Institute for the History of Medicine, 1983.

English-Lueck, J. A. *Health in the New Age - A Study in California Holistic Practices*, N.p.: University of New Mexico Press, 1990.

Family Recipe Book, Newcastle, Ont.: Northrop and Lyman, 1869.

Farmers' Directory and Housekeepers' Assistant Containing Recipes and Axioms Highly Useful to all Persons. Toronto: J. Cleland, 1851. Silverthorn Papers. Ontario Archives.

Fowke, Edith. *Folklore of Canada.* Toronto: McClelland and Stewart, 1976. Reprint, 1982.

Godfrey, Charles M. *Medicine for Ontario.* Belleville, Ont.: Mika Press, 1979.

Guillet, Edwin C. *Pioneer Settlements in Upper Canada.* Toronto: University of Toronto Press, 1933.

Holling, S. A., John Senior, Betty Clarkson, et. al. *Medicine for Heroes: A Neglected Part of Pioneer Life*. Erin, Ont.: Mississauga South Historical Society; Boston Mills Press, 1981.

Jefferis, B. G., and J. L. Nichols. *The Household Guide or Domestic Cyclopedia. Home Remedies for Man and Beast; A Complete Receipt Book*. 14th ed. Toronto: J. L. Nichols & Co., 1894. [20th ed., 1899]

King, Lester S. "Do-It-Yourself Medicine." *Journal of the American Medical Society*, 200 (1967).

Lacourciere, Luc. "A survey of folk medicine in French Canada." In *Explorations in Canadian Folklore.* Edited by Edith Fowke and Carole H. Carpenter, 237-252. Toronto: McClelland and Stewart, 1985.

Ladies of Toronto and Towns in Canada, comps. *The Canadian Home Cook Book.* Toronto: Hunter, Rose and Co., 1877. Reprint, Toronto: Ontario Reprint Press, 1970.

Leading Canadian medical men, comps. *The Family Physician or Every Man His Own Doctor.* Toronto: Hunter, Rose and Co., 1909.

Lyman, Henry M., H. Webster Jones, et al. *The Practical Home Physician & Encyclopedia of Medicine.* Guelph, Ont.: World Publishing Co., [188-].

Macdermott, H. E. *One Hundred Years of Medicine in Canada*, 1867-1967. Toronto: McClelland and Stewart, 1967.

M'Millan, Alexander. *Dr. M'Millans's Formulas and Domestic Guide*. Ohio, 1882.

Melendy, Mary M., M.D. *Ladies Home Companion*. Toronto: Linscott Publishing, 1901.

Mitchinson, Wendy and Janice D. McGuinnis, eds. *Essays in the History of Canadian Medicine. Toronto: McClelland and Stewart, 1988.*

Moore, R. *The Artizan's Guide and Everybody's Assistant, Embracing Nearly 4,000 New and Valued Receipts, Tables, etc.*, Montreal: Lovell, 1875.

Morley, P., and R. Wallis, eds. *Culture and Curing*. Pittsburg, PA: University of Pittsburg Press, 1979.

Naylor, C. David. "Rural Protest and Medical Professionalism in Turn-of-the-Century Ontario." *Journal of Canadian Studies*, 21 (1986).

Newman, John B. *The Home Doctor: or Family Manual*, Stratford: Vivian & Campbell, 1862.

Parker, Mrs. Eliza R. *Economical Housekeeping - A Complete System of Household Management.* Toronto: J. S. Robertson and Bros., 1886. CIHM 8841.

The People's Home Library: A Library of Three Practical Books. [The People's Home Medical Book; The People's Home Recipe Book; The People's Home Stock Book.] Cleveland: R. C. Barnum, 1916; Toronto: Imperial Publishing, 1920.

Pierce, R. V., M.D. *The People's Common Sense Medical Adviser in Plain English; or, Medicine Simplified.* 88th ed. Bridgeburg, Ont. and Buffalo, N.Y.: World's Dispensary Medical Association, 1921 [36th ed., 1895].

Practioner, A. *The People's Guide to Health, Prosperity, and Good Old Age, with Recommendations of Dr. J. W. Kermott's Medicines*. London, Canada West: Blackburn's Steam Press, 1855, Ontario Archives.

Riddell, William R.R. "Popular Medicine in Upper Canada a Century Ago." *Ontario History*, XXV (1929): 398-404.

Risse, G. B., R. L. Numbers, and J. W. Leavitt eds. *Medicine Without Doctors: Home Health Care in American History.* New York: Science History Publications, 1977.

Roland, Charles G., ed. *Health, Disease and Medicine - Essays in Canadian History*. [Toronto]: Hannah Institute for the History of Medicine; Clarke Irwin, 1984.

Rutty, Chris. "Patent Medicine and Popular Health in Ontario: Medicine, Pharmacy and the Development of Government Legislation, 1890-1908." History paper, University of Western Ontario, 1990.

Seaborn, Edwin. *The March of Medicine in Western Ontario*. Toronto: Ryerson Press, 1944.

Shryock, Richard H. *Medicine and Society in America: 1660-1860*, New York: New York University Press, 1960.

The Skillful Housewife's Guide. Montreal: Armour and Ramsay, 1848.

Smith, W. H. *Smith's Family Physician*, Toronto: Hunter, Rose, and Co., 1869.

Smith, W. H. *Family Physician.* Montreal: John Lovell, 1873.

Smith, W. L. *The Pioneers of Old Ontario.* Toronto: George N. Morang, 1923.

Stewart, Shuyler, Reverend. *The Canadian Herbal or Botanic Physician, comprising a variety of the Indian remedies and medicinal plants of this country*. Hamilton, 1851.

Taylor, Margaret, and Frances McNaught, eds. *The Early Canadian Galt Cook Book*. Toronto: William Briggs, 1898.

Wesley, John. *Primitive Physic: or An Easy Method of Curing Most Diseases.* London: Milner and Sowerby, [1780?].

George Whitehouse Collection. *Accounts and recipe books.* Regional collection. D. B. Weldon Library, University of Western Ontario, London, Ont.

Ye Old Miller's Household Book: Valuable Recipes in All Departments. Toronto: The Campbell Mills Flour Co., 1899. [McLeod, George J. *The Dominion Cook Book.*]

Young, Daniel. *Young's Demonstrative Translation of Scientific Secrets, or, A Collection of Above 500 Useful Receipts on a Variety of Subjects*. Toronto: Rowsell and Ellis, 1861.

Young, James Harvey. *The Toadstool Millionaires: A Social History of Patent Medicines in America.* Princeton, N.J.: Princeton University Press, 1961.

Vanalstine Papers. Family Papers from Prince Edward County, Ontario, 1800-1860. Ontario Archives.

About The Author

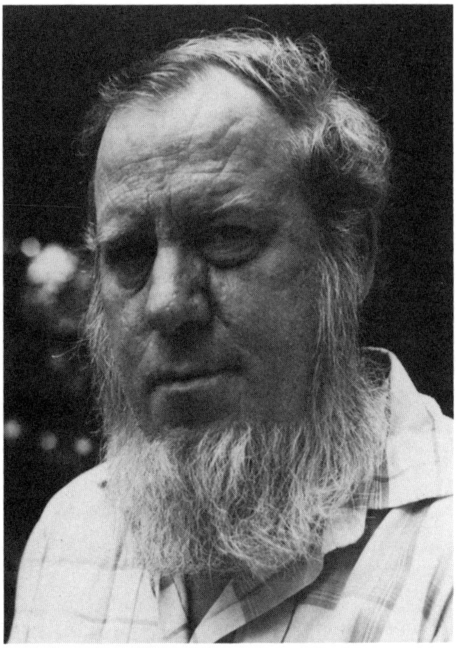

Photograph by G. B. Norcliffe

Notwithstanding the author's rather derelict appearance, he is generally viewed as being a friendly and positive person. Jim has always strongly denied the outlandish allegations that his costive mind has restricted what otherwise might have led to a balanced view of life.

Jim's interests include wandering in and out of 19th century Canada; "beavering away" in Kincardine at his pre-cut cord of firewood and contemplating the hypothesis that "a circle is a square that has faced reality."

Jim is an Associate Professor of Geography at Atkinson College, York University, and holds a BA (Hons) from the University of Western Ontario, a MSc from the University of Guelph and a PhD from the University of Glasgow, Scotland. He served as a councillor for 16 years in the town (now city) of Vaughan and lives in Kleinburg, Ontario.

For more copies of

Good for what Ails you

send $17.95 plus $4.50 to cover
GST, shipping and handling to:

GENERAL STORE PUBLISHING HOUSE
1 Main Street, Burnstown, Ontario
K0J 1G0

Telephone 1-800-465-6072
Fax 613-432-7184